Treating Phonological Disorders in Children

T0254696

This book is dedicated to our families and to the future

Look well therefore unto this day
for it is life
the very life of life
And in its path lie all
the realities and truths of existence.

Anon, ancient Sanskrit manuscript

Treating Phonological Disorders in Children:

Metaphon–Theory to Practice

Second edition

Janet Howell and Elizabeth Dean
Queen Margaret College, Edinburgh

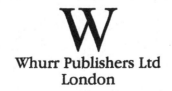

Whurr Publishers Ltd
London

© 1994 Whurr Publishers Ltd
First published 1991 by Far Communications
Second edition published by Whurr Publishers Ltd
19b Compton Terrace, London N1 2UN, England

Reprinted 1995, 1998, 2001 and 2004

British Library Cataloguing in Publication Data
A catalogue record for this book is available from the British Library.

ISBN: 1-897635-95-8

Photoset by Stephen Cary

Contents

Preface

The Metaphon approach to the remediation of disordered phonology in young children originated some ten years ago from our dissatisfaction with the management that was provided for this group of children. Therapeutic strategies did not appear to be responding to the growing understanding of the rule governed and predictable nature of disordered speech. Intervention often remained directed towards specific phonemes and the use of discrimination and production activities. Furthermore little attention appeared to be given to the learning situation in which therapy took place. Our attempts to respond to this situation have resulted in a treatment rationale that is targeted directly at the children's simplifying rules, using activities designed to bring about phonological change through enhancing knowledge of the phonological and communicative aspects of language, set within a therapeutic environment which maximises learning opportunities.

The first edition of this book gave us the opportunity to describe in detail the theoretical basis on which this therapy procedure was founded and to provide concrete examples of the possible organisation of intervention, together with suggestions for practical activities for clinical application. In this edition we have expanded and revised the original text to include more detailed discussions of aspects of the theoretical basis of the approach. In particular we have been able to include information about current investigations of the linguistic awareness of pre-school children. Because Metaphon is based on theoretical principles which are applied in therapeutic situations to meet specific client needs, rather than adhering to a rigid programme of predetermined activities, it can be adapted for use with different client groups, and children who speak languages other than English. As a consequence there has been considerable development in the application of Metaphon during the last four years and this edition gives us an opportunity to report on this development. To facilitate understanding of the vital importance of interaction between the child's response to the learning situation and the choice of therapy activities in Metaphon, week by week therapy planning and evaluation reports have been included in this edition. We hope that these will provide useful illustrations of how the approach is tailored to each child's specific learning requirements.

This book is intended both for readers who are new to the Metaphon approach and for those who have become interested in these ideas and methods through attending our workshops, listening to conference presentations or reading journal articles. In other words for those who wish to supplement their existing knowledge and for those who have not encountered this treatment method previously. For the latter, we have endeavoured to incorporate into the book practical guidelines which contain sufficiently detailed information to enable these readers, if they wish to do so, to plan and carry out Metaphon treatment systematically.

We are very grateful for the opportunity that Metaphon has given us to combine our interests in phonological disorder and the development of linguistic knowledge and learning. The fundamental responsibility for this treatment approach must rest with the authors but without the help and contribution of others the scope of this book would have been far more limited. First and foremost we would like to acknowledge the contribution of our Metaphon colleagues, Anne Hill, Daphne Waters and Jennifer Reid. The Metaphon assessment procedures represent the joint efforts of Daphne, Anne and ourselves. Anne treated the children in the first efficacy study and much of the data we use throughout the book is drawn from her very detailed and careful recording of her treatment sessions. The new section on treatment planning and evaluation would not have been possible without her meticulous observation and reporting. Daphne played a significant part in the early stages of the first efficacy study, and she continues to be an ardent supporter, with her research informing the Metaphon approach. We would like to thank her for her sound and welcome advice on the presentation and content of this edition. Jennifer is the Research Fellow working on the current efficacy study, we are very grateful for her outstanding academic and clinical contribution to the development of Metaphon and the enthusiastic help and encouragement she has given us in the preparation of this new edition.

Many of the recent developments in Metaphon come not from us but from other therapists who have become sufficiently interested in Metaphon to spend time applying it in ways other than in the original, one to one, therapy situation and to clients other than pre-school children with specific phonological disorders. Without their interest much of Chapter 9 would not have been possible. We would like to convey our very grateful thanks to the following therapists for taking time to give us information about their experience with Metaphon: Carolyn

Anderson, of Strathclyde University, and Julie Williams (now Tregonning) and her colleagues from the Paediatric Team of North Warwickshire National Health Service Trust, for information about using Metaphon in group treatment; Alison MacDonald of Queen Margaret College for sharing with us her experience of using Metaphon with hearing impaired clients; Kim Harland, Principal Speech and Language Therapist, North East Thames Regional Plastic and Burns Unit, for giving us detailed meticulous descriptions of her exciting and innovative use of Metaphon therapy with cleft palate children; Olwen Rees, Speech and Language Therapist, Gwynedd Community Health Unit, for her patience in explaining the complexities of the Welsh language to us and her verbal and written reports on her enthusiastic, but often frustrating, attempts to use Metaphon principles with Welsh speaking children. We would also like to thank our Swedish colleagues, Britt Hellquist and Britta Eriksson, and Angela van den Oetelaar of the Netherlands, for information about the use of Metaphon in their respective languages.

We hope that the figures and illustrations we have included in the book will facilitate understanding of the theoretical principles and practical application of Metaphon. We would like to thank Nigel Hewlett for permission to reproduce his model of speech production. Alistair Phimister drew the cartoon pictures for the phoneme test and the minimal pair pictures for pea and bee, and tea and key. Janet Sayles designed the referent cards for 'Mr Noisy/Mr Whisper' and those for the initial cluster reduction process. Cherie Rutter, Speech and Language Therapy Assistant, Thameside, drew the referent cards for 'Mr Nose/Mr Mouth'. Pictures such as these make an important contribution to the enjoyment of Metaphon therapy and we are very grateful to these artists both for interpreting our ideas so successfully and allowing us to reproduce some of their work.

In addition to those who have played a specific part in the compilation of this book we owe our thanks to many other colleagues and friends who have given us more general support and encouragement. We would particularly like to thank our current and former colleagues at Queen Margaret College, especially Professor Moira McGovern who gave us helpful advice and encouragement. We would like to thank our colleagues and fellow grant holders at the University of Edinburgh, Dr Morag Donaldson and Professor Robert Grieve, for their interest and support. The continuing evaluation of Metaphon would not have been possible without their help and that of the therapists who are currently participating in this investigation. We are very grateful to these clinicians for their good tempered and long-suffering responses to our stringent assessment and treatment requirements.

Finally, and most importantly, we thank the children who have taken part in Metaphon therapy sessions, and their parents. Their co-operation

and interest, children and adults alike, is boundless and without them
we would have little to write about. It is a great pleasure and privilege
to work with these children. We hope that this book will be of benefit
to them and help and encourage other therapists who work with them.

Janet Howell, Elizabeth Dean, Edinburgh, July 1994.

Chapter 1
Introduction

Over the last twenty years the practice of speech and language therapy has undergone radical changes. Nowhere is this more so than in the field of developmental language disorders where the contribution of linguistics has revolutionised assessment procedures. Authors such as Ingram (1976) and Grunwell (1981, 1987) have provided fundamental insights about the nature of developmental speech disorders leading to a new classification system. 'Dyslalia' is now long dead, and the use of the category 'developmental articulatory disorder' has given way to 'phonological disorder' which has in turn been modified to 'syntactic phonological syndrome'.

Yet again, the applied discipline of speech and language therapy has increased its knowledge base through research arising from other sciences; research which typically leads to a deeper understanding of the nature of the disorder. As clinicians, we are able to make a diagnosis of a linguistic disorder arising at the phonological level with more certainty and, further, to specify with accuracy the nature of the rule system operating. It is important to stress, however, that this is a symptom based diagnosis resulting from a description of the child's output phonology; we have no knowledge about the underlying nature and cause of the problem.

Without knowledge of the explanation of the disability we have to use what information we possess to determine an intervention strategy. We are responsible for planning and executing a remediation programme which will facilitate the child's shift towards the phonological system of his or her native language. In this endeavour the insights from clinical linguistics are vital but they are not sufficient. They tell us the target but not the route, the aim but not how we achieve it. How can children effect change in their phonological system? Do we have any theory that will inform intervention?

Disciplines such as psychology and, indeed, linguistics provide insights which clinicians have drawn upon to enhance therapeutic procedures but no fully developed theory of intervention is reported in the literature. We believe that speech and language therapists, with their unique combination of skills, have a major role to play in developing theories of intervention for linguistic disorders. It is arguable that only they are in a position to synthesise knowledge from several fields, including clinical practice, to create a viable theoretical underpinning for remediation. That such a theoretical framework is sorely needed is indisputable. Speech and language therapy is under growing pressure, both economic and theoretical, to justify its value. Without a stated and replicable therapeutic regime, efficacy studies are impossible. Without detailed studies of intervention there can be no increase in knowledge about sound clinical practice.

This argument can be illustrated by an outline of the growth of Metaphon therapy (Dean and Howell, 1986; Howell and Dean, 1987). Over ten years ago we stood in the Demonstration Clinic, at Queen Margaret College, and watched a young child through a one way mirror. Careful assessment had led to a diagnosis of severe phonological disorder and therapy had commenced; as was common at that time, this involved minimal pairs. The child was motivated, and interested in the games laid out for his amusement, but his phonological system was proving immovable, as we observed what was obviously his attempt to try to comply with what appeared to be the therapist's wishes. Having recently been interested in metamemory, we began to wonder about 'metaphonology', asking ourselves the question 'What do children know about sounds?' In the intervening years we have scoured the literature and questioned children in our pursuit of knowledge about their ability to think about and manipulate sounds.

This book represents not the end point in that search, but at least a resting point along the way. In Chapters 4, 5 and 6 we discuss in detail the linguistic and psychological theoretical frameworks we have adopted for our approach to remediation. The discussion of language and learning in these chapters is not presented in isolation but is closely related, at all times, to Metaphon therapy so that we can illustrate how the theoretical basis influences practical application.

In line with our belief that the therapy programme should be stated clearly so that it can be replicated, Chapter 7 is concerned with the practical organisation and application of Metaphon in the clinic and provides detailed examples of the activities employed at each stage in therapy. This chapter also contains detailed case records which chart session by session planning and record the therapist's impressions of response to therapy and how she modified activities in subsequent sessions to overcome the child's problems.

In Chapter 8 we put our ideas to the test. This chapter is concerned with two studies which investigated the effectiveness of Metaphon. The chapter presents what we believe is positive evidence for the change effected by remediation and, as a useful adjunct, gives information about organisational factors such as phonological change effected over a specific time span.

All treatment must be preceded by assessment of the client's strengths and limitations in order that these can be precisely targeted for optimum therapeutic effectiveness and efficiency. This book mirrors this maxim by devoting Chapters 2 and 3 to discussions about current knowledge and assessment of phonological disorder.

In Chapter 9 we look at the wider applications of Metaphon and describe the way in which the principles which underlie Metaphon therapy can be applied to children with different characteristics and needs, learning in diverse situations. The book concludes with a brief final chapter which outlines possible future developments of Metaphon.

It is appropriate that we finish this introduction with the caution that we have given on every occasion when we have talked and written about Metaphon therapy. Our initial aim was to explore the literature to ascertain what insights we could gain which would inform our therapy for phonologically disordered children. We then assembled what we had read, together with our clinical experience, into a framework to guide the planning and execution of remediation. We occasionally say that this is a 'philosophy' but that dignifies this framework beyond its actual significance. What we have, and what we present here, is a collection of notions which we believe can profitably be taken into account when devising an intervention programme.

The looseness of this description is intentional. Our aim was to utilise current theories of language and learning in our therapy for phonological disorder. We present the theories that we drew upon and try to support our framework for remediation. However, if we go further and lay down a specific therapeutic programme we are defeating our purpose. Metaphon aims to be an approach sufficiently flexible to be applicable to and adaptable for individual children with all their inherent variability. Following its guidelines will allow therapy to be replicable but at all times to be specifically planned for individual children. Metaphon is not inviolable, or even static. It is constantly changing to take account of new insights which come from the literature, discussion with colleagues and from the children and parents themselves.

We trust that this book will be interesting for clinicians and that, whilst it does not necessarily suggest radical departures from current practice, some passages will provoke thought. If we could listen and watch we would hope to hear such comments as 'That makes sense. It is almost what I do. I wonder if...'

Chapter 2
Current Knowledge of
Phonological Disorder

Efficient therapeutic planning depends upon a clear understanding of the nature of the problem that requires remediation. In this chapter therefore we will look at what is currently known about phonological disorder and consider the implications of this knowledge for therapeutic intervention in general and the Metaphon approach in particular. Space does not allow for more than a general overview but we will provide appropriate references for readers who would like to look at any topic in more depth.

First of all we will review the evidence which leads us to accept the proposition upon which Metaphon therapy is based; that phonological disorder is a developmental language learning disorder rather than an articulatory production problem (Gibbon and Grunwell, 1990). Then we will consider briefly the extent to which the problem is confined to the phonological aspects of language and examine what is known about the causes and explanation of the disorder. (See also Gibbon and Grunwell (1990).)

Phonological Disorder – A Language Learning Problem

The following quotation from Grunwell encapsulates what would now be accepted by many clinical linguists and speech pathologists and therapists as the essential nature of phonological disorder:

> a linguistic disorder manifested by the use of abnormal patterns in the spoken medium of language (Grunwell, 1981: p. 9).

We will consider what this definition means in a little more detail.

Children who are learning to talk have to master two main tasks. They have to learn how to articulate a number of different speech sounds and they also have to learn how to contrast and combine these sounds to produce meaningful pronunciation patterns. In other words they have to know how to integrate features of voice, place and manner to physically produce phonetic segments and they have to acquire the rules of adult language which determine how these segments are organised to form words. A diagnosis of phonological disorder is based on descriptive analysis which demonstrates problems in this second aspect of learning to talk. Children who are labelled as phonologically disordered have failed to make the same progression in learning adult pronunciation rules as children of the same age who are developing normally.

Satisfactory explanations for delay in acquiring adult phonological rules remain elusive and we are probably dealing with a spectrum of possible influences. One of the main questions centres around the relationship between phonetic developmental aspects of learning to talk and phonological rule acquisition, a point to which we return after we have looked at the children's rule systems.

It is said that instead of using adult pronunciation patterns phonologically disordered children have their own individual rule systems. But what do we mean by this? In this context rules are descriptions of the relationship between a child's speech patterns and the patterns of the adult language. We are able to derive, from such descriptions, the exact nature of a child's pronunciation patterns (Hewlett, 1990). From writing rules of this kind we know that the pronunciation patterns of phonologically disordered children are usually systematic, that is, the children are likely to be consistent in the way they realise adult targets. The following example provides an illustration. A child may produce both 'tea' and 'key' as [ti], that is the contrast between these two words is collapsed. The systematic predictable nature of the child's pronunciation patterns becomes apparent when further investigation shows that the problem is not confined to these two words. Usually children who substitute /t/ for /k/ at the start of 'key' will make the same substitution whenever they encounter a word that starts with /k/, and they may also use /d/ instead of /g/. As a result intelligibility will be reduced, unless we can guess from the context or have become familiar with their rule system over time.

The example we used, the collapse of contrast between alveolar and velar stops, is labelled 'fronting'. Strictly speaking the use of labels of this kind means we are referring to rule types rather than individual rules, because such a rule may be applied differently by different children. For instance it may operate only word initially or in all word positions, or may be used for a whole class of sounds or only one sound. This point is well illustrated by the examples we use in Chapter 3.

The essential point to remember is that phonologically disordered children primarily have consistent patterns of pronunciation which are different from those of the adult language. That is they have their own set of realisation rules and it is possible to work out and write down these rules from listening to samples of the children's speech. From these rules we can then predict how a child is likely to pronounce an individual word and state how this pronunciation differs from adult pronunciation.

Most of the rules phonologically disordered children use are also used by normally developing younger children, but phonologically disordered children persist in using them over a much longer time span. Phonologically disordered children may also use rules which have been termed 'idiosyncratic' or 'atypical'. These are rules which appear to be unique to a specific child or which have only been recorded infrequently, and then not usually in the speech of normally developing children. Initial consonant deletion would be regarded as an atypical rule. Children using this rule will delete some or all consonants word initially; as a consequence 'cat', 'bat', 'fat', etc., would all be realised as [at].

Each phonologically disordered child will have his or her own unique combination of rules. These may be developmental rules only, or a combination of developmental and atypical rules. Children may use only one or two rules or as many as thirteen or fourteen. The extent to which a rule type is applied also varies between children, as we saw above. Some will have obligatory rules, and for others the same rule will be optional, that is it may apply in some situations but not others. To recap, using our examples, the child who fronts velars may do so in all word positions or only word initially. A child who deletes consonants at the start of words may delete all consonants, only stop consonants or only voiceless stop consonants. At the end of this chapter we look at the general therapeutic implications of this rule governed behaviour and in Chapter 3 we provide data from children in our own clinic which demonstrates the variation that occurs among children's rule patterns. More information about typical rule patterns can be found in Stoel-Gammon and Dunn (1985).

We have said earlier that a diagnosis of phonological disorder is based on an analysis and description of the children's pronunciation patterns rather than on a demonstrated difficulty in articulating the speech sounds of their native language. The predictable nature of the children's pronunciation patterns reinforces the notion that we are concerned with a linguistic/cognitive disability. We cannot, however, rule out the possibility that there may be a phonetic component influencing phonological rule development. Linguistic analysis shows that many, but not all, phonologically disordered children have restricted phonetic inventories; that is, some adult sounds may not appear at all in a particular child's speech sample. (An account of the phonetic characteristics of phonologically disordered children can be found in Stoel-Gammon and Dunn (1985).) On the other hand we should also remember that many phonologically disordered children are frequently able to imitate sounds that they do not use spontaneously. They may also use such sounds contrastively in some word positions but not in others. That is, the sound is part of their phonetic inventory but is not fully exploited. Thus we cannot automatically presume that the child is unable to articulate the sounds he or she does not use.

The relationship between phonetic development and rule simplification is a complex issue (see Hewlett, 1990). To reduce it to a simple dichotomy between articulating, and using, sounds is a gross simplification. Our current position on this issue is that we would not rule out the possibility that some children who have a diagnosis of phonological disorder may have difficulties in physically producing some sounds. Others may lack knowledge of how to produce certain segments, that is they may not yet have grasped how to combine specific features say of place and manner to make a particular sound (Hewlett, 1990). In Metaphon we can adjust therapy to overcome possible weaknesses in speech processing. Consequently an essential part of our total assessment procedure assesses children's ability to imitate sounds in isolation, in nonsense syllables and words.

We can therefore summarise the preceding discussion by arguing that Grunwell's definition of phonological disorder highlights the belief that the disorder arises essentially from a difficulty with learning and applying the phonological rules of adult language rather than from a difficulty with articulatory production. In other words we are suggesting that phonological disorder is essentially a phonemic/organisational problem rather than a phonetic/production difficulty. It is this concept of the disorder that underlies and determines the Metaphon approach to treatment.

As we have seen, evidence to support a linguistic conceptualisation of phonological disorder comes from interpretation and analysis of speech samples, that is, such inferences are drawn mainly from descriptive evidence. Although such analysis is invaluable in revealing the specific nature of the children's difficulties it does not tell us **why** some children have these problems. This conceptualisation of the problem as a linguistic disorder also raises questions about **where** the breakdown originates in the phonologically disordered child's organisation and production of speech. We will examine these points shortly, but before doing so we will consider what is known about the other aspects of the language abilities of phonologically disordered children.

Other Language Abilities of Phonologically Disordered Children

Until recently it has been customary to assume that the linguistic difficulties of phonologically disordered children are confined to the phonological aspects of language. Grunwell (1981), for example, uses adequate comprehension and expressive language abilities as defining characteristics in her detailed examination of the disorder. With the increased availability of a large range of formal language assessments and the increased use of a variety of linguistic analysis techniques we are able to examine and compare ability at all levels of language in much more detail. As a result the assumption of a specific phonological problem has been increasingly questioned. Current thinking is reflected in the growing tendency of some authors to use the term 'syntactic phonological syndrome', to refer to children who have predominantly phonological difficulties (Rapin and Allan, 1983; Bishop and Rosenbloom, 1987). Whether or not we choose to use this term, the available evidence suggests that it is probably most constructive to consider phonological disorder as part of a spectrum, or continuum, of developmental language disorders. Some children will have, as far as can be determined, a specific phonological disorder, and our experience suggests that this is still the majority of the total population of language disordered children. Other children will have phonological problems with accompanying motor planning or motor execution difficulties. And some children will have more generalised language difficulties, to varying degrees, of which phonological difficulty will form only one aspect. (See Bishop and Edmundson (1987) for further general discussion on this point.)

Recent studies which have examined the relationship between phonological disorder and other language abilities have been carried out by Smit and Bernthal (1983), Edwards et al. (1984) and Shriberg et al. (1986). These studies show that for many children phonological problems occur alongside other language difficulties, but they tell us little about the nature of the associations between different language abilities. Whether for example some other, underlying, factor may affect several levels of language, or alternatively, whether there is some cause and effect relationship between different levels of language. It is possible that impairment at one level may interact with and disturb other levels of language. Different aspects of language may make competing demands during attempts to communicate. If, for example, there is an attempt to use a complex grammatical structure the child may consequently lose precise control of articulation at the phonetic level (Panagos, Quine and Klich, 1979; Hambrecht and Panagos, 1980). It is important to bear this possibility in mind when planning therapeutic activities. Crystal (1987) and Schwartz (1991) provide detailed discussions of the relationships between co-occurrence of language deficits and the interaction between different levels of language during on line processing.

Before leaving the topic of linguistic characteristics we also have to consider the possible effect of the phonological disorder on the child's communicative inter-relationships. We have to take into account how the communicative partners' efforts to understand what the child is saying may influence how they respond to the child and how, in turn, this might affect the child's more general linguistic processing abilities. Gibbon and Grunwell (1990) have some comments to make on this point. They suggest that because phonologically disordered children are difficult to understand they may be provided with inadequate responses which will not encourage language development. They go on to make the suggestion that children who become aware of their communicative problems may also avoid communicative interchange. Gardner (1989) is researching the parental responses of phonologically disordered children and we refer to the relevance of her work to treatment strategies in Chapters 5 and 6 of this book.

What then are the implications of the association between phonological and other language disabilities for treatment? Phonological problems, whether they occur in isolation or as part of a wider spectrum of language disorders, are disadvantageous to children. They require specific therapeutic attention and constitute a significant challenge to speech therapists. Metaphon is an appropriate intervention strategy for isolated phonological disorder. It may also be an appropriate therapeutic method for treating disordered phonology when it is part of a wider language disability, or when it occurs in conjunction with motor planning and motor execution constraints. In these latter instances Metaphon can be combined with other remediation strategies, but the basic principles of Metaphon are such that it can be adapted to a variety of client groups (see Chapter 9).

Why do children have problems with the phonological aspects of language? We will look at this question from two perspectives. First we will consider factors in the child's developmental history and environment that may influence phonological development. After this we will adopt a simple speech processing approach and consider those investigations which have attempted to discover weaknesses in the child's perception, processing or production of speech.

The Search for Causative Factors

Investigations which have looked for overt causes of phonological disorder have either searched for correlations between phonological development and other factors, such as hearing loss, or have compared the characteristics of phonologically disordered and normally developing children to isolate factors which appear to predominate in the disordered population. Shriberg et al. (1986) provide a useful discussion of the extensive literature on this topic. Shriberg and his colleagues isolate over one hundred possible causative factors; these range from histories of hearing and feeding difficulties to reduced cognitive abilities and factors such as parental attitudes.

It is not surprising given the wide range of possible causative factors that studies of this type usually indicate that there are associations between some developmental and environmental factors and phonological disorder. For example, Shriberg found that about half of 160 children that he investigated had a history of hearing problems, most often characterised as middle ear infection. We should be very wary of putting too much dependence on the results of studies of this kind, however. For instance, developmental factors such as middle ear infection are not confined to the phonologically disordered population and the significance of some factors apparently associated with phonological disorder is not known. Conversely there may be subtle differences between phonologically disordered and normally developing children which have not yet been identified because methods of measurement may be insufficiently sensitive.

The investigation of possible causative factors is, as we can see, inconclusive and beset with difficulties. For most of these children it will not be possible to attribute their problem to a specific cause. But for maximum effectiveness of Metaphon therapy it is desirable that we take into account possible developmental and environmental influences on the child's disorder and adapt our therapeutic activities accordingly. We would therefore stress that therapists should continue to search for such possible explanations when assessing individual children.

Speech Processing Explanations

As well as looking for overt causes of phonological disorder we can examine speech perception, processing and production and try and determine any weaknesses along this continuum which may contribute to the child's phonological difficulties. In other words we also adopt a psycholinguistic approach to investigate possible explanations of phonological disorder. A framework for the psycholinguistic investigation of developmental speech disorders in the clinical situation can be found in Stackhouse and Wells (1993). We will look first at the auditory discriminatory and oral motor aspects of speech processing. After this we will consider the few investigations which have addressed the cognitive aspects of speech processing, that is how children might mentally store and organise words or phonemes.

Auditory Discrimination Abilities

Investigations of these abilities are extensive, and the results are equivocal; see Winitz (1969), Grunwell (1981) and Bird and Bishop (1992) for detailed reviews. Following an evaluation of the available literature Gibbon and Grunwell (1990) conclude that there is:

> a tendency for children with developmental articulation disorders to display difficulties in performing auditory discrimination tasks. This is especially evident in children with more severe speech disorders (Gibbon and Grunwell, 1990: p. 138).

This statement reflects the situation for the phonologically disordered population as a whole and as such directs us towards an aspect of behaviour that we should investigate in attempting to explain the problem. It does, however, hide the fact that the individual investigations have very divergent results and that some investigators failed to find any association between auditory discrimination and phonological disorder; see for example Supple (1983) and Howell (1989). More importantly, most of the investigations which demonstrated a group tendency towards poor performance in auditory discrimination also found wide variation of ability within groups of phonologically disordered children. The simple response to the lack of consistency between and within investigations is to conclude that we are concerned with a heterogenic population and that poor auditory discrimination may explain phonological disorder for some children but not others.

Unfortunately this inference, although probably correct, is not the only factor we have to consider. Determining the true position about the role of auditory discrimination skills in explaining phonological disorder is more complex. We have also to take into account the methodological differences between studies. First, different studies are probably looking at different populations; the severity of the disorder is not usually specified and criteria for subject selection vary. Second, there are variations in the tasks used to assess this ability. These may make different cognitive demands on subjects and may be assessing different aspects of auditory discrimination. See Locke (1980) for a detailed critical discussion of methods used to assess auditory discrimination.

Even if it were possible to resolve methodological difficulties, we cannot assume that any demonstrated auditory discrimination difficulties are responsible for the production problems. Winitz (1969), for example, suggests that perceptual problems may result from, rather than cause, the phonological difficulties.

Finally we do not know whether the tasks used in these experiments actually assess the type of discriminatory abilities that are required for phonological acquisition. It should also be remembered that auditory discrimination is a very complex phenomenon and that activities such as the frequently used same/different judgements of minimal pair words provide a rather crude, general assessment of it. For instance sounds can be distinguished on a multiplicity of acoustic cues (Strange and Broen, 1980) and it is not possible to determine which of these are being employed to carry out the task. It is also possible that some children may have discriminatory difficulties which are too subtle to be discovered by the use of minimal pair tasks. In short, auditory discrimination differences may exist between phonologically disordered and normally developing children which are not being discovered by methods currently available in the clinical situation. Simply employing more sophisticated experimental techniques does not solve the problem, however. Comparison of investigations using synthetically generated phonemes and syllables, a situation which provides experimenters with opportunities to control for the multiplicity of variables within speech signals, also reveals inconsistent findings (Bird and Bishop, 1992).

What then are the clinical implications for this lack of certainty in determining possible relationships between auditory perceptual ability and phonological disorder? If we are to provide the most effective and efficient therapy for these children it is essential that we discover more about the relationship between auditory discrimination and phonological ability. In particular we need to look in more detail at the skills that are required to carry out different types of auditory discrimination tasks and how such skills may be related to speech output.

We are in no doubt that speech therapists should continue to include investigation of auditory discrimination ability in their assessment battery for phonologically disordered children. We should, however, look very closely at the assessment methods we are using and include consideration of what cognitive skills are required to carry out each task when interpreting results.

The first requirement is that we should be examining each child's discrimination ability in relation to the contrasts that are neutralised in their own speech. This will mean devising specific target items for each individual child. More general assessments of auditory discrimination are unlikely to provide the specific information that is required.

We should then consider the nature of the cognitive processing that different tests require. Locke (1980) provides detailed information about various types of auditory discrimination tasks and Stackhouse and Wells (1993) show how these tasks can be used as part of a psycholinguistic investigation. For instance, same/different judgements of minimal pair words can be made on the basis of acoustic information held in short term memory. In contrast, tasks in which pictures depicting minimal pairs are used and the subject is asked to point to the picture of one of the pair of words when spoken by the tester, require subjects to access their internal representations of the words. Difficulty at either, or both, of these levels might have an influence on phonological development. It is only by carrying out tests that can identify precise levels of breakdown that we can increase our understanding of phonological disorder and provide precisely targeted intervention. We believe that the routine application of minimal pair auditory discrimination activities in treatment is of little value unless the child demonstrates a specific inability to discriminate between phonemes. Metaphon therapy activities do include matching and categorising sounds, listening for similarities and differences and discriminating between classes of sounds. Such tasks require the children to discriminate between phonemes but this is only one aspect of such activities, as we shall demonstrate in Chapter 6.

We have described two aspects of auditory discrimination but Bird and Bishop (1992) suggest that it is not sufficient for children to be able to tell sounds apart, they should also be able to categorise sounds; that is, recognise that a sound, for example /s/, in different word contexts belongs to the same phoneme despite variation in acoustic and articulatory qualities. This ability to categorise sounds depends on being able to discriminate between sounds but it also depends on other factors; it raises questions about auditory memory and theories about the way that sounds and words are represented and stored in the mind. These are questions that we will return to when we have considered the oral motor characteristics of phonologically disordered children.

Oral Motor Characteristics

We have already said that most phonologically disordered children appear to have little difficulty in articulating speech sounds. The oral motor ability of phonologically disordered children has also been assessed by tests of oral form perception and by non-speech oral repetition tasks. In oral form perception tasks (or oral stereognosis) small shapes are placed in the subject's mouth and they are asked to name them or to match them with pictures of the shapes (Deutsch, 1984). Oral repetition (or diadochokinesis, DDK rates) measures the speed at which subjects can repeat strings of stop consonants. Such tasks are believed to be appropriate measures of orosensory and oromotor ability which affects articulatory programming and tactile and kinaesthetic feedback. It has been hypothesised that this may be inadequate in phonologically disordered children (Gibbon and Grunwell, 1990).

Some phonologically disordered children have been found to perform more poorly than normal children on such tasks. But, as with the perception tasks, it is not possible to come to firm conclusions about cause and effect relationships. Stoel-Gammon and Dunn (1985) for instance point out that the phonologically disordered child's inability to speak normally may be a disadvantage in such tasks. These authors conclude that a proportion of such children may have some kind of motoric immaturity or deficiency. Abbs and Kennedy (1982) also suggest that some phonologically disordered children:

> may not have the normal capacity to develop sensorimotor control and thus cannot learn the intended reactions necessary for executing certain linguistic rule processes consistently.(Abbs and Kennedy, 1982:p. 104.)

No empirical evidence to identify the nature of this deficit has been obtained from measuring DDK rates or from carrying out oral form perception tasks. However, instrumental investigations such as acoustic studies of speech timing and variability and electropalatographic investigations do provide evidence which suggests that some phonologically disordered children have problems at the level of motor implementation. For instance a recent study by Waters (1992) involving spectrographic measurement and perceptual analysis of multiple token data from phonologically delayed children, normal children and adults lends some support to the view that speech motor co-ordination may be less mature in phonologically disordered children than in normal children of the same age. In particular, mean speech rate was significantly lower in the disordered group when measured in segments per second over multiple repetitions of a phrase (Dean et al., in press).

These recent investigations lend further support to the view that children labelled as phonologically disordered are not a homogeneous group and that individual children's difficulties in realising adult pronunciation rules may result from a variety of possible underlying deficiencies. It follows therefore that children will have different therapeutic needs. We believe that different children might benefit in different ways from taking part in Metaphon therapy and that this form of intervention can be adapted to meet the needs of several diverse groups. This would include providing opportunities for some children to develop their speech motor skills, but this would still be done without direct focus on sound production (Dean et al., in press). In Chapter 9 we provide some practical examples of how this might be done.

We will turn now to the link between perception and production and consider whether any aspects of what is known about the way words and sounds are stored in the brain help us to understand the nature of phonological disorder.

Mental Representation

We are using the term mental representation to cover both short term memory for reception and processing of language and long term storage.

The short term auditory memory ability of phonologically disordered children has received relatively little attention. The few investigations that have been carried out tend to use serial digit recall tasks. The results from these investigations are inconclusive. For instance, Howell (1989) found no significant difference between the performance of a group of phonologically disordered children and a matched group of children with normally developing phonology on the auditory sequential memory section of the Illinois Test of Psycholinguistic Abilities (Kirk, McCarthy and Kirk, 1968). On the other hand Henry (1990) reported a significantly poorer performance by 'severely speech disordered' 3–5 year old children compared with normally developing children of similar age. This result should be treated with caution, however, because it is doubtful whether Henry's subjects are representative of the phonologically disordered population as a whole.

A more general consideration with regard to these investigations is the question of whether the ability to recall digits is an appropriate method of assessing phonological memory. We do not know whether the ability to remember digits taps into the same cognitive processes that are required for remembering and sequencing speech sounds. A more appropriate approach may be to carry out investigations of this aspect of memory within the working memory model proposed by Gathercole and Baddeley (1993). One aspect of this model is a phonological loop which processes and maintains phonological information. It consists of a phonological short term store and a sub-vocal control process used for rehearsing and recoding information into phonological form. Gathercole and Baddeley suggest that children from the age of 4 appear to retain auditory information within the phonological loop and use a rudimentary form of rehearsal.

It is possible to speculate about how such a process might have a role in establishing appropriate adult pronunciation targets. Work is currently being carried out by Elizabeth Dean investigating the relationship between output phonology and phonological memory using nonword repetition tasks, the customary way of assessing phonological memory within this theoretical model, and we await the results with interest. Meanwhile Gathercole et al. (1994) found that language disordered children aged between 7 and 9 were poorer at repeating nonwords than a control group of children matched for non-verbal skills and a younger control group matched on verbal skills. The language disordered children performed at the level of 4 year old children and the deficit in phonological memory was greater than the deficit on other linguistic skills that were tested.

Gathercole argues that these findings suggest that a deficiency in phonological working memory is one of the main causes of word learning difficulties in children with impaired language development. However Snowling, Chiat and Hume (1991) argue that non-word

repetition tasks may also be affected by other factors such as perception and difficulty with assembling appropriate articulatory patterns.
Researchers are becoming more skilled at devising assessments which
can measure discreet aspects of speech and language processing, such
as the instrumental measures of perception and production we
referred to earlier in this chapter. As a consequence it will become
increasingly possible to isolate factors which may be contributing to a
child's linguistic difficulties. The working memory approach offers
exciting possibilities for extending the investigation of disordered
phonology. If phonological memory ability is found to be associated
with phonological acquisition we look forward to the time when
appropriate tests of phonological memory become a part of the routine
assessment of children with disordered phonology. Having considered
the potential role of short term, or working memory, in phonological
processing we now need to look at how phonological information
might be stored in the brain for access for phonological production.

Phonological Representation

The manner in which words are stored in the brain is usually referred
to as underlying, lexical or phonological representation. If, as we are
advocating, phonological disorder is primarily a phonemic organisational problem and our aim is to create change in phonological output,
it is particularly important that we should consider the possible nature
of storage and planning processes.

Research has demonstrated quite clearly that there are some differences in the way that children and adults store words. Aitchison and
Chiat (1981) for instance suggest that full phonological representation
may not be achieved before the age of nine. Aitchison (1987) provides
an excellent discussion on this topic. Knowing that there are differences between child and adult representations enables us to suggest
that these differences may be associated with or influence phonological
development in some way. However, we know of no work which has
specifically suggested that there may be differences between normally
developing and phonologically disordered children's phonological
storage and processing.

Unfortunately these processes are not directly accessible to investigation so hypothetical models or theories have to be constructed about
possible organisational patterns on the basis of observable behaviour.
In the following paragraphs we describe the basic outlines of some suggested developmental and speech processing models, examine their
validity and discuss how they might be of use in the clinical situation.
The main differences between the developmental models we describe
centres around the nature of perception and storage.

Smith (1973) suggests that the young child in the process of phonological development has adult like perception and a single mental store of representations which match the adult form. If this model is accepted then presumably failure to achieve adult pronunciation must result from motoric limitations. A conclusion which, as we have already discussed, may not be appropriate for most phonologically disordered children.

An alternative theory is suggested by Macken (1980). She suggests that very young children may have incorrect perception and a single store of incorrect representations. But it is difficult to accept this possibility in the light of the well known tendency of both normal and phonologically disordered children to reject their own forms as incorrect when they are imitated by others or played back to them on a tape recorder. This is known as the 'fis phenomenon', after a description by Berko and Brown (1960) of a normal child's rejection of an adult's imitation of the child's pronunciation of 'fish' as [fis].

This evidence of some unwillingness by children to acknowledge their own production of a word, combined with failure to achieve the adult pronunciation of the word, is, however, compatible with a third possibility. This suggests that younger normally developing children and phonologically disordered children have adult like perception but store words as simplified forms of the adult targets (Ingram, 1976; Waterson, 1981). We saw earlier in our discussion of perceptual abilities that there are many parameters by which words can be recognised; it is therefore possible that words can be stored in a simplified form. The stored form may contain only some of the features of the adult target, these may be sufficient to allow rejection of a perceived form but not sufficient to allow the child to reproduce exactly the adult target.

Waterson (1987) provides a theoretical model of the development of phonological representation which is compatible with this third option. Waterson uses her model to explain mismatch between perception and production and to account for pronunciation changes during the process of normal phonological development. The model provides a detailed account of the manner in which child representations may differ from adult representations and the way in which these representations change and develop. Two levels of mental representation are proposed. One level consists of a store of possible phonetic patterns without meaning, which are responsible for reception and recognition of speech. The second level is a store of lexical phonological patterns, which have both phonetic specifications and meaning; these are responsible for interpretation and production. According to Waterson the child starts with neither of these levels and development is dependent upon increasing perceptual and memory ability and is concerned with the process of recognising and matching auditory patterns. The representations are constructed and reconstructed on the basis of the maximum perceptual information available to the child at any one time.

A fourth possibility which accounts for mismatches between perception and production, and also proposes that the child has two representations is suggested by Straight (1980). The two representations in this model are a perceptual representation matching the adult form and a production representation matching the child's own pronunciation form. In other words an input and an output lexicon. This is a more straightforward and economical model than Waterson's in that it can be used without needing to make any presumptions about possible perceptual limitations. This model is given support by Chiat (1983) who argues that the only way to account for differences between perception and production (at least in one phonologically disordered child that she studied) is to posit input and output lexicons. Further information about some of these models of lexical representation can be found in Dinnsen (1984) and Stoel-Gammon and Dunn (1985).

The concept of an input and output lexicon has also been used by Hewlett (1990) as a basis for constructing a model of single word processing activity in children. We believe that this model has a significant contribution to make in helping us to examine both the nature of phonological disorder and the process of effective intervention. We will therefore describe it in some detail.

The model proposes syllable and segmental level motor processing components which are responsible for putting together the required sequences of articulatory gestures for the production of single words (Figure 1). Two alternative routes to the Motor Processor are suggested, a faster automatic route direct from the Output Lexicon and another slower route from the Input Lexicon via the Motor Programmer.

It is envisaged that the Input Lexicon contains the perceptual features of a word. When these features are received by the Motor Programmer it attempts to devise a motor plan for the execution of the word. When this plan is finalised it is passed to the Motor Processing component and subsequently realised via the Motor Execution component. When a plan for a particular lexical item is judged to be satisfactory its articulatory feature specification is entered into the Output Lexicon. This specification is then available to be directly accessed by the Motor Processor for subsequent production without access to the Motor Programmer. In other words the Input Lexicon via the Motor Programming route to the Motor Processor enables children to create motor plans for new words, whilst the Output Lexicon via the Motor Processing route provides for rapid execution of familiar motor plans.

The motor plans that are established in the Output Lexicon may not of course match the adult target. If this is the case, revision is achieved by re-accessing the Motor Programmer to devise new motor plans. In the course of normal development revision probably takes place spontaneously as a consequence of listeners' responses to the child's communication attempts. Persisting non-adult realisations in the

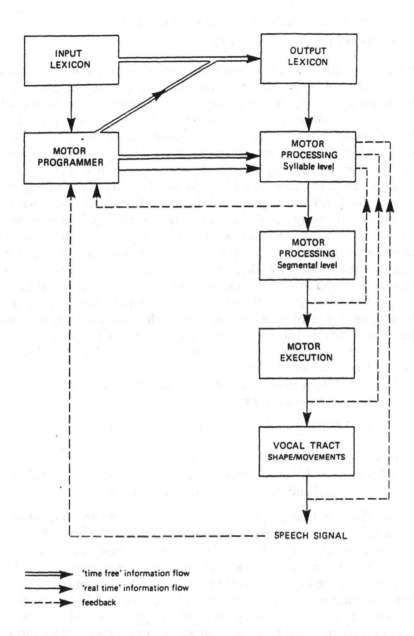

Figure 1 A model of speech production (from Hewlett, 1990, with permission)

speech of the phonologically disordered child are a clear demonstration that for these children automatic revision does not take place. We will use Hewlett's model below, and in Chapter 6, to help us explain how Metaphon therapy encourages children to make the changes that are needed.

Therapeutic Implications of Mental Representational Models

We have seen that there are several theories about the possible organisation of lexical representation and planning during the process of phonological development and we have suggested that some models stand up to examination better than others. We have taken some time to consider these purely hypothetical possibilities because we believe they have important therapeutic implications. The essential aim of therapeutic intervention must be to bring about phonological change. We would suggest that examining phonological disorder within the framework of these models helps us to understand what processes we are attempting to change and assists in making therapeutic strategies explicit. In other words such models can help therapists to specify exactly what they wish to achieve in treatment and how they aim to bring this about. We have already mentioned the use of a dual representational model by Chiat (1983) and that the Waterson model could also be useful for speech therapists in the analysis of speech output and the prediction of possible patterns of change. An example of the utilisation of theoretical models in the discussion of therapeutic intervention, with particular reference to the Hewlett model, can be found in Howell and McCartney (1990).

Hewlett (1990) suggests that at least the following four conditions must be met for revision of a rule:

1. Awareness of the insufficiency of current production.
2. A desire to change it.
3. Knowledge of the relevant crucial articulatory targets.
4. Sufficient dexterity of the vocal apparatus to implement articulatory targets at speed and in a variety of phonetic contexts.

You will see in later chapters when we come to describe the theoretical basis and the practical application of Metaphon therapy how we fulfil these conditions. Briefly we believe that bringing about a desire for change can be achieved through the therapeutic activities we use which are designed to excite and motivate the child. Knowledge of the crucial articulatory targets is developed by giving the child opportunities to explore the contrasting features of speech sound categories. Opportunities to 'play' and 'experiment' with non-speech and speech sounds may enhance speech production. Awareness of insufficiency of current sound production is brought about through positive feedback about a child's communicative competence in the later stages of Metaphon therapy.

If we relate these strategies to the Hewlett model we can see that enhancing a child's awareness will alert the child to the need to make a revision to the pronunciation of a word. This can only be done by re-accessing the word from the Input Lexicon and producing it by the slow route, that is via the Motor Programmer. For example, the child who fronts velars will habitually pronounce 'key' as [ti], the result of accessing the established, but inappropriate, motor plan from the Output Lexicon. Increasing awareness of required adult targets will encourage the devising of a new motor plan via the Motor Programmer which will lead to the pronunciation of 'key' as [ki]. Activities which are used in Metaphon therapy to provide the child with opportunities for exploring and experimenting with sounds may provide an increased knowledge base which facilitates this process. If the child is given the opportunity to experiment and practise within a therapeutic framework which provides appropriate interpersonal feedback and encourages self monitoring the relevant rules will be gradually revised. This will bring about the replacement of the old motor plan with an appropriate adult like representation in the Output Lexicon that will be available for automatic access and use.

Children's performances in experiments which are designed to assess knowledge of language, linguistic awareness, are also contributing to the discussion about the possible nature of children's mental representations of words. All reports of investigations that require children to match rhyming words, or segment the phonemes in a word, describe consistent differences between the abilities of phonologically disordered and normally developing children. Linguistic awareness forms the basis of our treatment procedures and the results of this type of treatment suggest that using activities which are designed to develop metalinguistic ability also accelerates change in phonological development. We discuss the theoretical aspects of linguistic awareness in more detail in Chapter 4 and cover practical application in Chapter 6.

In this chapter we have been concerned with current knowledge about phonological disorder. We have put forward arguments to support the view that it is a developmental language disorder, we have examined the relationship between phonological and other language problems and looked for explanations of the disorder with reference to overt causes and speech processing activity, and we have considered the therapeutic implications of these last points. We will end the chapter by summarising the therapeutic implications of the proposition that phonological disorder is a developmental language disorder.

Therapeutic Implications of a Linguistic Interpretation of Phonological Disorder

The adoption of a linguistic orientation to phonological disorder has therapeutic implications both in terms of planning the order of remediation and the nature of that remediation. Detailed analysis of the child's speech output should be an essential preliminary to therapeutic planning whatever treatment methods the speech therapist favours. Such analysis enables the therapist to determine, and state explicitly, what features require remediation and in what order such remediation might be most beneficially provided. Thus such treatment progression will be based both on what the analysis reveals about the individual rule governed behaviour of each child and how this relates to what is known about phonological acquisition in general. For example, analysis will show the extent to which a child's simplifying rules are developmental or idiosyncratic, in other words, common to normally developing and other phonologically disordered children or exclusive to an individual child. In the latter case more detailed decision making and unique therapeutic activities may be required. Analysis will also reveal the extent to which the operation of each process is obligatory or optional. In other words a process may affect all sounds within a class and all positions within a word, or affect only certain positions in word structure, or certain sounds within a class. On the basis of this information the therapist may, for instance, decide to work on an optional process at the start of treatment. By doing this the therapist will assist the child to generalise an adult pronunciation pattern, that is already in use, to other areas of production.

These analysis procedures, together with more general information about the child's interests and background are an essential preliminary to providing Metaphon therapy. In Chapter 3 we look in detail at the analysis procedures we use. Employing data from children we have seen in our own clinic we will demonstrate how analysis determines detailed individual therapeutic planning for each child.

A linguistic interpretation of the disorder also has implications for remediation strategies, the activities that are used in treatment. Such an interpretation suggests that intervention should be focused on finding ways of encouraging children to extend the range of contrasts between the sounds they use, rather than on the production of single phonemes. It suggests that therapists should be helping children to eliminate the simplifying phonological rules they are currently using and adopt instead the rules used by the adults in their environment. In other words it implies that remediation should be concerned with developing children's knowledge of the structure and organisation of their native language rather than with the production and practice of phonetic segments.

Grunwell (1983) suggests:

> changes in speech production need to take place not so much in the mouth but in the mind of the child. The aim of treatment is to effect cognitive reorganisation rather than articulatory retraining (Grunwell, 1983: p. 167).

Metaphon is designed to facilitate such cognitive reorganisation through utilising and developing the children's metalinguistic awareness, and we will show how this is translated into practice in Chapter 6.

Chapter 3
Linguistic Assessment of Phonological Disorder and Metaphon

In the previous chapter we said that speech therapists must have information about the precise nature of the children's pronunciation patterns to enable them to plan the most efficient treatment programmes. In this chapter we look in a little more detail at the analysis of phonologically disordered speech and describe the Metaphon Resource Pack (MRP) (Dean et al., 1990) and the procedures we have devised to assist in this analysis procedure. We will then use data collected from our own subjects to demonstrate how phonological analysis informs treatment planning. Before we do this we will describe the typical characteristics of phonologically disordered speech.

Phonologically Disordered Speech

According to Grunwell (1981) the phonetic characteristics of phonologically disordered speech include the following: a restriction in the number and variety of phonetic segments, restriction in the range of feature combinations with rare use of fricatives, (with these usually confined to one place of articulation), frequent absence of affricates and the phonotactic structure of syllables tending towards simple consonant vowel (CV) or consonant vowel consonant vowel (CVCV) forms. Stoel-Gammon and Dunn (1985) draw together the findings of several published studies and show a similar picture of simple syllable shapes and restricted sound systems. They add that the size of the phoneme inventory of the typical phonologically disordered child is usually about half that of the adult inventory. These authors also found that some of the individual data samples also contained one or two non-English phonemes.

In the previous chapter we gave some examples of typical phonological rules used by phonologically disordered children. We will now look in a little more detail at the range of pronunciation patterns that have been noted in data collected from these children. These rules are described in terms of 'simplifying phonological processes'. There are, of course, other procedures available for analysing children's speech, but process analysis has proved a particularly useful method of description on which to base intervention programmes. Process analysis is derived from the theory of Natural Phonology proposed by Stampe (1979). This theory was originally formulated as an explanation of normal phonological development but it has increasingly been used to describe patterns of disordered phonology. There are theoretical points about the precise difference between rules and processes, but these need not concern us here. It is sufficient to say that a process is essentially a rule type and in the last chapter we defined a rule type as a rule which can be applied to varying extents across a class of sounds or different word positions. The examples we present later will make this point clear.

Stoel-Gammon and Dunn (1985) used process analysis to compare the findings of eight different investigations containing the data from 128 phonologically disordered children aged between 2;8 and 13 years. They found that nine simplifying processes occurred more frequently than any others. These were: three structural simplifying processes – consonant cluster reduction, final consonant deletion and unstressed syllable deletion; four substitution processes – stopping, fronting of velars and palatals and liquid simplification; and two sound change processes – assimilation and voicing.

As well as these commonly occurring processes, processes which incidentally are also found in the pronunciation patterns of younger normally developing children, there was also evidence of many other processes in the data and, as we remarked in the previous chapter, considerable intersubject variation in the type and frequency of occurrence of particular processes.

Data reported from two studies of Scottish children (Moss, 1985; Howell, 1989) shows very similar patterns to those described by Stoel-Gammon and Dunn. Moss looked at the phonological processes of 15 phonologically disordered children aged between 3;7 and 6;6. She found that all these children used a selection of all the processes observed in normal children and that these occurred more commonly than unusual or non-normal processes. But all her subjects exhibited between one and seven processes not normally found in normal development. Backing of alveolar stops to velar place of articulation was particularly common, appearing in the data of 11 of the children.

Howell (1989) investigated 21 children with disordered phonology, whose ages ranged from 3;8 to 5;5. All 21 children reduced initial consonant clusters and 19 fronted velar stops. In addition they all demonstrated between one and three atypical processes but these were very variable in type and occurrence.

When our current efficacy study is completed (see Chapter 8), we will have data for 50 phonologically disordered children. Identical collection and analysis procedures have been used to obtain this data from each child and when the investigation is complete the data will provide an invaluable source of information about the type and extent of pronunciation patterns of phonologically disordered children. The first data returns in this investigation suggest that they will confirm the results of other studies in relation to both the extent and type of processes that are in operation.

In this description of pronunciation patterns we have referred to developmental processes, that is those that have been observed in younger normal children, and processes which have not been reported in this group; these are termed variously, 'atypical', 'abnormal' or 'idiosyncratic' processes. The distinction between normal and atypical processes has sometimes been used to postulate two groups of phonologically disordered children, 'delayed' and 'deviant' (Leonard, 1973; Ingram, 1976). It has also been used as a criterion for determining whether or not to provide intervention and there is a tendency to suggest that deviant processes may be resistant to treatment whilst developmental processes will resolve spontaneously; see, for example, Dodd and Iacano (1989).

We do not believe that this is a particularly useful distinction to make within the context of Metaphon therapy. The data cited above shows that most phonologically disordered children have a combination of developmental and atypical processes. It is possible to divide processes into groups but not to sub-divide the children on the basis of their presenting processes. Distinguishing between delayed and atypical processes is not a primary focus for us when planning treatment and we have found that, although it is not always easy to find labels for atypical processes, they may respond to therapy with the same speed as developmental processes.

Having outlined the kind of speech patterns we might expect from this group of children we will go on to describe the analysis techniques we use to determine the pronunciation patterns of individual children, an essential preliminary to planning therapy. But first we will say a little about data collection.

Data Collection

A comprehensive speech sample is an essential first step towards a satisfactory analysis. This may seem to be stating the obvious, but the usefulness of the subsequent analysis is largely dependent on the type and extent of the data on which it is based. Full instructions for collecting and transcribing speech samples can be found in Phonological Analysis of Child Speech (PACS) (Grunwell, 1985). We will just make brief reference to the type and amount of data that we consider constitutes an adequate sample for therapy planning purposes.

First, it is advisable to have information about the child's pronunciation from both connected speech and single words, for analysis and comparison. Single word data will give us information that can easily be replicated on subsequent occasions, and in general terms might perhaps be said to represent the child's best efforts. There is no guarantee, however, that the child's ability to pronounce single words will be matched in spontaneous connected speech, the medium of normal communication, so we also want to know about pronunciation ability in this situation.

Second, the size of the data sample is also important. Grunwell (1985) suggests that a sample of 200–250 words should be the aim. She says that this size of sample is large enough to contain the child's realisations of most adult targets more than once so that any significant variability is revealed. We would agree with Grunwell that a comprehensive sample is required to determine the precise nature, and extent, of a child's phonological difficulties. However, collecting and analysing a sample of this size, although desirable, is extremely time consuming. This is compounded by the fact that young children often have a short attention span and a limited vocabulary. The Metaphon Resource Pack was specifically designed to respond to the dilemma of the need to provide detailed information within an economical time frame.

The Metaphon Resource Pack

The MRP is designed to provide a phonological assessment which gives the therapist in-depth information about a child's pronunciation abilities without the need for extensive administration and analysis time. We have found that it will provide sufficient information for planning therapy for the vast majority of phonologically disordered children. In a very few children with very complex or variable systems it may be necessary to use the MRP data to carry out other analysis procedures.

In common with many other phonological assessments the MRP uses process analysis to examine the nature of children's pronunciation patterns. Process analysis is currently the most commonly used system for profiling disordered phonology and the one that we have found to be most useful when planning Metaphon therapy. There are, of course, many other possible analysis procedures but it is beyond the scope of this volume to provide an account of these. Information about other procedures and their advantages and disadvantages can be found in Grunwell (1985 and 1987). Although we favour process analysis for clinical purposes we are, of course, not discounting the value of other analysis procedures and their accompanying theoretical models. We are for instance currently investigating the use of therapy activities based on the work of Bernhardt (Bernhardt and Gilbert, 1992) who uses non-linear phonological theory to investigate phonologically disordered speech.

Process analysis is a particularly useful clinical procedure because it has a developmental perspective and is suitable for analysing both normal and disordered phonological development. It can therefore be used to make comparisons between a child's actual and expected level of phonological development. This facility for comparing the phonologically disordered child's pronunciation patterns with normal pronunciation development helps the therapist to decide whether treatment is required and to determine the most appropriate order of treatment. This type of analysis will also reveal whether the processes the child is using are confined to developmental processes or include atypical (unusual or idiosyncratic) processes. This information may have a role in determining the order in which treatment is provided and will alert the therapist to the need to design specific therapeutic activities.

In addition to the MRP several other analytical frameworks based on process analysis are available; see, for example: Grunwell (1985, 1987); Hodson (1980); Ingram (1976, 1981); Shriberg and Kwiatkowski (1980); Weiner (1979). There are strong similarities between these frameworks although they may use different terminology or classify and organise the processes in slightly different ways. The terminology that is used in the MRP to describe processes is closest to that of Grunwell (1985, 1987).

The MRP provides opportunities for the detailed examination of nine systemic and four structural simplifying processes. Systemic simplification processes are those where essentially one consonant is substituted for another, for example fronting. Structural simplification processes are those where the structure of a word or syllable is changed, for example cluster reduction. The processes examined by the MRP are listed in Table 1.

We have selected for specific attention those processes which, according to the literature and our clinical experience, occur most frequently in phonologically disordered speech. The assessment includes processes which are universally recognised as developmental such as fronting and those which have only rarely been reported in the developmental literature, and might therefore be termed atypical processes, for example initial consonant deletion. Table 1 shows the age by which developmental processes are expected to disappear during the process of normal development. It is important to point out that the ages given for process elimination are very general approximations and that variations of six months either way can be expected in normal development (Grunwell, 1985).

It is essential that users of the MRP should examine the child's data for any evidence of the use of simplifying processes other than those we have specifically singled out for attention and analysis. In the interests of economy we have specifically focused on those processes which

Table 1 Simplifying phonological processes assessed by the Metaphon Resource Pack

Process	Approximate age of suppression
Systemic	
Velar fronting	3.00 to 3.06
Palato-alveolar fronting	4.00 to 4.06
Stopping of fricatives	
/f/	2.6 to 3.00
/v/	3.00 to 3.06
/θ/	2.06 to 3.00 → fronting to '[s] type'
/ð/	3.06 to 4.00 → fronting to [d] or [v]
/s/	2.06 to 3.00
/z/	3.00 to 3.06
/ʃ/	2.06 to 3.00 → fronting to '[s] type'
Stopping of affricates	3.06 to 4.00 → fronting to [ts; dz]
Backing of alveolar stops	(atypical process)
Syllable final devoicing	3.00 to 3.06
Syllable initial voicing	2.06 to 3.00
Liquid glide simplification	4.06 →
Dental fronting	4.06 →
Structural	
Initial consonant deletion	(atypical process)
Final consonant deletion	3.00 to 3.03
Intial cluster reduction/deletion	3.06 to 4.00
Final cluster reduction/deletion	(not available)

Notes:
Approximate age of suppression = the age at which these processes have ceased to be used, or are used inconsistently, by most children of this age.
Atypical process = a process that is not recorded in normal acquisition data.
Not available = a process reported in normal acquisition but where no age of suppression is given

our clinical experience suggests occur most frequently in phonological-ly disordered speech, but it is a simple matter to look for and record the occurrence of other processes and the MRP analysis sheets provide spaces for doing this. Investigation beyond these most commonly occurring processes is required because all children, although they have strategies in common, have their own unique way of coping with learning the pronunciation patterns of their native language. This means that no finite group of processes exists; consequently it is not possible to design an assessment package to specifically investigate all possible processes.

A particular feature of the MRP is the provision of a quantitative scoring procedure, from which a percentage occurrence can be calcu-lated. Percentage occurrence of processes is rarely calculated in other published assessment packages. However, we believe quantitative measures are essential for effective clinical decision making; without them we cannot make accurate assessments of phonological change. We also require information about the extent to which a process is operating to determine whether it constitutes a hindrance to the child's communicative effectiveness and consequently whether it should be a target for therapy. We know that there are considerable differences in the extent to which simplifying processes are used by individual children. For example, Dunn and Davis (1983) analysed the frequency of occurrence of a number of common simplifying processes in the data of nine phonologically disordered children. These authors found that although most of the processes they investigated occurred in the speech samples of all their subjects, the extent to which they were used by each subject varied greatly. It is also of interest to note here that, with one exception, speech samples collected from 21 normally developing children, aged between 3;6 and 5;5 with EAT (Edinburgh Articulation Test) Standard Scores of 100 or above, all contained examples of some simplifying processes (Howell, 1989). With the exception of the fricative simplification process (/θ;ð/ → /s;z/), none of the processes were operating at a high level of occurrence. Nevertheless 13 of these children exhibited some cluster reduction and a similar number some palato-alveolar fronting.

The MRP is divided into three sections: a Screening Procedure, Process Specific Probes and a Monitoring Procedure. This three stage approach to data collection and analysis was our solution to the need to reconcile the competition between requiring a comprehensive speech sample and the demands upon speech therapist's time. Decisions about what simplifying processes should be targeted at the start of a course of therapy are based on the results of the Screening Procedure followed by the administration of the Process Specific Probes. The Monitoring Procedure is designed to assess the extent and pattern of change during a programme of therapy. This procedure enables the therapist to quantify therapeutic progress and from this to determine when to cease providing treatment for a particular process. Further details of this procedure can be found in Chapter 8.

The Screening Procedure is designed to provide an overview of the simplifying processes occurring in the child's speech. A single word sample is collected using a picture naming task, or if desired by a combination of picture and object naming. The sample consists of 44 monosyllabic core words and 26 more complex words. The 44 core items provide several opportunities to note the occurrence of common simplifying processes in word initial and word final positions. The 26 additional items are intended for the investigation of within word consonant realisations and to aid the identification of additional processes. The tester is also advised to encourage the child to talk about the pictures so that realisations of the words in connected speech can be collected for comparison with the single word items. All the items have been chosen to be within the expressive vocabulary of 3;6 to 5 year old children.

The child's responses are transcribed on to a data collection sheet (see Figure 2) and if possible checked from a tape recording.

The design of the analysis sheets that are provided with the Screening Procedure (Figure 3) enables the therapist to assess the occurrence of each simplifying process in turn by a quick and easy process of transferring transcribed words from the data collection sheet into the appropriate section of the analysis sheet. The occurrence of

Data Collection Sheet

Name:_____ Clinician:_____ Date:_____

Ref no.*	Item	Transcription	Ref no.	Item	Transcription
1	cup		23	jam	
2	gun		24	house	
3	knife		25	path	
4	sharp		26	door	
5	fish		27	smoke	
6	kiss		28	bridge	
7	sock		29	train	
8	glass		30	chair	
9	watch		31	red	
10	nose		32	spoon	
11	mouth		33	plane	
12	yawn		34	fly	
13	leaf		35	sky	
14	thumb		36	sun	
15	foot		37	wing	
16	toe		38	splash	
17	snake		39	tent	
18	van		40	salt	
19	fast		41	crab	
20	girl		42	sweet	
21	stairs		43	sleeve	
22	big		44	zip	

*Ref no. refers to the pictures in the Screening Assessment Picture Booklet.

Figure 2 Data Collection Sheet, Screening Procedure, Metaphon Resource Pack (from Dean et al., 1990, reproduced by permission of NFER-NELSON Publishing Company Limited, Darville House, 2 Oxford Road, Windsor SL4 IDF. All rights reserved.)

each process is then converted into an error score. This error score provides an initial indication of the nature and extent of the child's use of simplifying processes and forms the basis of a more intensive examination of potential problems using specifically selected Process Specific Probes. The whole process of administering and analysing the Screening Procedure should not take more than about thirty minutes in total.

The Process Specific Probe material consists of a set of stimulus pictures and record sheets for each of the 13 simplifying processes. The items used for each probe provide in-depth information about the operation of the relevant process by including all the phonemes which may be affected by that process in a variety of phonetic environments and syllable positions. For example, there are 19 items for each of the velar and palato-alveolar fronting processes and 46 items to cover five different types of initial cluster reduction/deletion.

The decision on which of the probes to select for administration is based on the qualitative and quantitative information derived from the Screening Procedure. We suggest that any process which is operating at 50% or greater occurrence in any syllable position should automatically be probed. This numerical guideline is only the starting point in the decision making process. In those instances where the Screening Procedure contains only a small number of items assessing a particular process it is advisable to administer a probe if there is any evidence of the process operating in the child's data. We also need to examine all the collected data alongside the quantitative information. For instance it is possible that percentage occurrence of a process may sometimes conceal rather than reveal a particular problem. We can illustrate this with an example: the occurrence of initial consonant deletion. In the interests of economy only six words are selected for analysis for this process in the Screening Procedure, and only two of these are fricatives, even though initial consonant deletion is frequently restricted to fricatives. Scrutiny of the data collection sheet will, in this example in particular, quickly reveal additional information which will influence which probes should be applied.

The data collected in the Screening Procedure should also be used to determine whether there is any occurrence of processes other than the 13 we have selected for specific attention which require further investigation. The stimulus pictures in the Process Specific Probes provide an excellent source of material for constructing probes for investigating additional processes and it is rarely necessary to look for stimulus material beyond the MRP.

We stress the need for a careful examination of the child's data sample because it is inevitable that there will be some loss of information at a surface level in any assessment instrument where practicality and time constraints are an important consideration. The design of the MRP,

Analysis Sheet

Occurrence of systemic simplifications

Velar fronting

	Syllable-initial			Syllable-final	
Ref no.*	Item	Occ.	Ref no.	Item	Occ.
1	cup		7	sock	
6	kiss		17	snake	
2	gun		22	big	
20	girl		37	wing	
	TOTAL	/4		TOTAL	/4

Stopping of fricatives

	Syllable-initial			Syllable-final	
Ref no.	Item	Occ.	Ref no.	Item	Occ.
5	fish		13	leaf	
15	foot		11	mouth	
14	thumb		6	kiss	
7	sock		38	splash	
36	sun		43	sleeve	
4	sharp		10	nose	
18	van				
44	zip				
	TOTAL	/8		TOTAL	/6

Palato-alveolar fronting

	Syllable-initial			Syllable-final	
Ref no.	Item	Occ.	Ref no.	Item	Occ.
4	sharp		5	fish	
30	chair		9	watch	
23	jam		28	bridge	
	TOTAL	/3		TOTAL	/3

Stopping of affricates

	Syllable-initial			Syllable-final	
Ref no.	Item	Occ.	Ref no.	Item	Occ.
30	chair		9	watch	
23	jam		28	bridge	
	TOTAL	/2		TOTAL	/2

/θ/ → /f/

	Syllable-initial			Syllable-final	
Ref no.	Item	Occ.	Ref no.	Item	Occ.
14	thumb		11	mouth	
			25	path	
	TOTAL	/1		TOTAL	/2

Context-sensitive voicing

	Syllable-initial				
Ref no.	Item	Occ.	Ref no.	Item	Occ.
25	path		5	fish	
16	toe		14	thumb	
6	kiss		36	sun	
			4	sharp	
				TOTAL	/7

Backing of alveolar stops

	Syllable-initial			Syllable-final	
Ref no.	Item	Occ.	Ref no.	Item	Occ.
16	toe		15	foot	
39	tent		42	sweet	
26	door		31	red	
	TOTAL	/3		TOTAL	/3

Liquid/glide simplification

	Syllable-initial				
Ref no.	Item	Occ.	Ref no.	Item	Occ.
9	watch		12	yawn	
13	leaf		31	red	
				TOTAL	/4

Word-final devoicing

Ref no.	Item	Occ.	Ref no.	Item	Occ.
41	crab		43	sleeve	
31	red		10	nose	
22	big		28	bridge	
				TOTAL	/6

*Ref no. refers to numbers on the Data Collection Sheet.

Figure 3 Systemic Process Analysis Sheet, Screening Procedure, Metaphon Resource Pack (from Dean et al., 1990, reproduced by permission of NFER-NELSON Publishing Company Limited, Darville House, 2 Oxford Road, Windsor SL4 IDF. All rights reserved.)

however, ensures that a considerable amount of readily accessible data is automatically collected for further scrutiny if required, and we encourage all users to look beyond the quantitative information to obtain a detailed picture of a child's pronunciation difficulties.

Before we go on to the therapy planning procedure using the MRP we need to say something about examining the phonetic features of the child's speech.

Phonetic Analysis

There are various aspects to a phonetic analysis such as the phonetic inventory, the phonetic distribution, the range of clusters and the range of syllable types used by the child. Of primary importance to this discussion is the range of sounds the child has in his or her speech, in other words the phonetic inventory. The data collected for phonological analysis can be used to compile this. In addition we want to know which sounds, not represented in spontaneous speech, the child is able to imitate, allowing us to build up a picture of potential motor processing constraints (see Chapter 2 and below).

There are a variety of ways of representing a phonetic inventory. The chart presented as Figure 4 illustrates a simple method of presenting information about the child's consonant inventory.

	LABIAL		DENTAL		ALVEOLAR		POST-ALVEOLAR	PALATAL	VELAR		GLOTTAL
NASAL		(m)				(n)				(ŋ)	
PLOSIVE	(p)	(b)			(t)	(d)			k	g	
FRICATIVE	f	(v)	θ	ð	s	z	ʃ	ʒ	x		h
AFFRICATE							(tʃ)	dʒ			
APPROXIMANT	ʍ	(w)				(ɹ)		ɹ	(j)		
TRILL						(r)					

Figure 4 Consonant inventory (Sue, chronological age 4;2)

The chart is used to record the child's consonant inventory by circling those consonants that appear in the child's data sample. Any use of non-English sounds can also be recorded on the chart by writing them in the appropriate section of the grid. It is a very simple matter to examine the child's data sample and record information in this way. We have illustrated the use of the inventory in Figure 4. We can see at a glance from this table that Sue has a restricted consonant system, she uses only one English fricative, voiced bilabial /v/, and she has no velar plosives. It is important to point out that all the consonants that are present in the child's speech sample, not only those that are used appropriately, will be recorded on such a chart. It is then possible to determine what speech sounds are available to the child when planning which processes to target. (More extensive information about recording and analysing phonetic characteristics can be found in PACS (Grunwell, 1985).)

We have made no mention of vowel sounds so far and most investigations of the speech sound characteristics of disordered phonology have focused on consonants. Vowels can sometimes present problems for phonologically disordered children, see Reynolds (1990) for a report of a detailed study. If difficulties with vowels are apparent from the child's speech these should be noted and analysed; Reynolds provides information which will be useful in this respect. We have successfully treated collapse of contrast between vowel sounds, but we have not carried out any systematic investigation of the use of Metaphon for vowel system abnormalities.

Having discussed the assessment of phonologically disordered speech we can now describe how phonological analysis is a vital aspect of treatment planning and illustrate some of the points we have made above by looking at data from some of our own phonologically disordered clients.

Clinical Decision Making

Before we describe the individual children it is perhaps appropriate to provide a brief reminder of the general considerations which influence the choice of processes for treatment.

The chronological age of the child should be taken into account. As we saw earlier there is a large variation in the age at which developmental processes are eliminated from children's speech. Care should be taken to make sure that processes which are selected for treatment are not those which are still reported as being prevalent in normally developing children of the same age as the child referred for therapy. As a general rule processes which are said to be eliminated earliest in normal phonological development are usually treated before later resolving processes.

In some instances it may be appropriate to capitalise on any spontaneous change that may be occurring in the child's speech. Variable use of a simplifying process and the adult target in a particular syllable position may be evidence of change. Syllable initial use of a process may indicate change, such as when the child usually fronts velars but realises them correctly in the context of a following back vowel.

The intelligibility of a child's speech is another criterion which is frequently suggested for determining therapy targets. Judging intelligibility can be a rather subjective process but there does seem to be some general agreement about the relative effect of different types of simplifying processes on listener understanding. For instance, syllable initial voicing is probably less disruptive than stopping of fricatives and atypical processes may be more disruptive than persisting normal processes.

It is also appropriate to utilise information from a phonetic inventory about the sounds that are available to the child. For example a child may have velars in word final position but not elsewhere. Some children may be able to imitate sounds in isolation that they do not use in speech. We have suggested that a simple imitation task where the child is asked to repeat sounds in isolation or with a following vowel should be an essential part of assessment. The consonant inventory chart we described earlier can be used to record the child's responses.

To summarise, decisions about what simplifying processes to target will depend primarily on each child's unique pattern of processes but factors such as chronological age, variability of processes, potential effect on intelligibility and what speech sounds are available to the child will exert an influence on the order in which we target processes.

We will now use data from seven of the children who participated in the first efficacy study to illustrate the different combinations of simplifying processes used by phonologically disordered children and demonstrate how we make decisions about planning a course of therapy. We have divided this illustration into two parts. In the first section we provide an overview of the data from four children with very different phonological profiles and large variations in the outcome of therapy. For these four children we describe the decision making process for therapy planning, outline the outcome of therapy and speculate on the factors that affected the outcomes for each of the children. In the second lot of case reports we look at a further three children with different degrees of severity, in terms of the number and type of simplifying processes they use, in rather more detail and discuss similarities and differences between them.

We start our discussion of the first four children at the stage when Process Specific Probes have been administered, listing the number of simplifying processes with a percentage occurrence of over 50% with regard to a particular syllable position or class of sounds. For example, we have considered syllable initial velar fronting separately from velar fronting in syllable final position and we have distinguished between a process of initial fricative/affricate deletion and a process of initial deletion of stops/approximants for ease of comparison.

It is not customary in Metaphon therapy to plan the focus of the programme of therapy beyond making a decision about which will be the first one or two processes to be targeted because we have found that Metaphon therapy frequently results in generalisation of phonological change to processes that have not been directly targeted. Consequently it has not been found to be particularly useful to make rigid plans in advance for ordering the targeting of all the child's processes. Our regular monitoring of change throughout remediation ensures that therapy can be targeted most economically where it is likely to have greatest effect.

Example 1

David was 4;1 at the start of therapy. He was the youngest of four boys. Developmental milestones were normal and there was no significant medical history. Language comprehension and vocabulary level, as measured by the Reynell Developmental Language Scales (RDLS) (Reynell, 1977) and British Picture Vocabulary Scales (BPVS) (Dunn et al., 1982) respectively, were above average. In addition to phonological problems he was also noted as having a fast rate of speech, unusual intonation patterns and some hyponasality. He presented with a relatively large number of simplifying processes; these are listed below.

Velar fronting	syllable initial and final
Stopping of fricatives	syllable final
Stopping of affricates	syllable initial and final
Liquid/glide simplification	syllable initial
Initial consonant deletion	fricatives and affricates
Initial consonant cluster reduction	fricative + consonant.
Final consonant cluster reduction	

At the age of 4;1 David was an obvious candidate for treatment. He had a wide range of simplifying processes both structural and systemic and one of the structural processes, initial deletion of fricatives and affricates, is an atypical process.

There were several possible targets for the start of therapy. It is perhaps easiest in this case to say first which processes would not be a priority. Liquid/glide simplification is still appearing in the speech of some normally developing children at this age. Stopping of affricates would not be targeted before stopping of fricatives as it is a later resolving process and we would also hope for a generalisation effect from targeting stopping of fricatives. Similar possibilities apply to consonant cluster reductions.

We were left with three principal targets for the start of therapy: velar fronting (syllable initial and final), stopping of fricatives (syllable final),and initial consonant deletion (fricatives and affricates). An examination of his consonant inventory showed that there was no evidence of velar plosives in his data and he used only one English fricative /v/. He also used the non-English palatal fricative /ç/ and the glottal plosive /ʔ/. His imitation skills were relatively poor, and he was unable to imitate /k;g;s;z/ although he could imitate other fricatives.

A decision was made to target velars (word initial) first in the expectation that there might be generalisation to word final position without further therapy. Work on initial consonant deletion, of fricatives and affricates, would follow. This second process was chosen for targeting for two reasons. First, initial consonant deletion can be a very disruptive process in terms of intelligibility and second, if a child acquires the ability to produce fricatives in initial positions, this may then be generalised to replace stops in word final positions.

Velar fronting in word initial position was targeted for 10 sessions and resulted in gradual elimination of the process from that position, but contrary to our expectations there was no immediate generalisation to elimination in word final position. Therapy was then switched to initial consonant deletion, fricatives were targeted word initially for 10 sessions. This resulted in establishing fricatives word initially with spontaneous generalisation of affricates, but there was no spontaneous carryover to the elimination of word final and within word stopping of fricatives or affricates, although some spontaneous drop in consonant cluster reduction was noted.

This first period of therapy had not resulted in as much generalisation as might have been expected; David was still fronting velars, although only word finally, stopping fricatives and affricates word finally and still reducing some clusters. He had made considerable progress but this tended to be restricted to what had been specifically targeted. He was given a further period of 12 sessions of therapy and progress was reviewed ten months after his first assessment. At that time David had a phonetic problem of interdental /s/ and /z/, possibly accounted for by the lack of two upper front teeth. Gliding of /l/ was restricted to /sl/ clusters and /θ/ was realised as [f] and there was some glottal insertion before final fricatives. Although these remaining phonological problems were very minor the therapist reports that he could still be difficult to understand at times. Other factors such as a fast rate of speech, unusual intonation and hyponasality probably contributed to this occasional unintelligibility, which David usually overcame without difficulty when a listener asked for clarification.

The main feature of David's response to therapy was the relatively small amount of generalisation that occurred. With hindsight it is possible to speculate, looking at his rather poor imitation skills and the additional features we noted about his speech, that his phonological problems resulted, at least in part, from motor processing constraints. The question of modifying Metaphon activities to respond to possible individual difficulties of this kind is taken up again in Chapter 9.

However, we conclude that the choice of processes to target was entirely appropriate in David's case.

Example 2

Ruth was 3;7 at the start of therapy. She was the second child of three. Her developmental milestones were normal and there was no significant medical history. Her language comprehension, as measured by the RDLS, was above average, and she had a slightly below average vocabulary score.

Ruth presented with the following simplifying processes:

Velar fronting	syllable initial
Stopping of fricatives	syllable initial
Stopping of affricates	syllable initial
Liquid/glide simplification	syllable initial
Initial consonant cluster reduction	plosive + consonant
Initial consonant cluster reduction	fricative + consonant

These are all developmental processes, and the systemic processes are only operating in word initial position and she is using the adult target in other positions. As she was only 3;7 with a relatively straightforward phonological profile she would not be a high priority case for intervention. She was, however, given a course of treatment; a decision that was influenced by the fact that Ruth had all the English consonants in her phonetic inventory, but was not exploiting them fully. There was no evidence of any non-English sounds and she had excellent imitation skills.

There were two obvious but competing targets for therapy in Ruth's case, fronting velars and stopping fricatives. She had both velars and fricatives in her sound system and both processes are eliminated at approximately the same age in normal development so deciding which process to target first was fairly arbitrary.

In the event fronting of velars was targeted first, for nine sessions. By this time, despite a rather slow start and a tendency to get bored with activities very quickly, the process was resolved and she was making spontaneous corrections in connected speech. Seven sessions targeting fricative stopping (word initially) followed. This resulted in successful elimination of the process and spontaneous generalisation to stopping of affricates and considerable elimination of cluster reduction.

Ruth was then put on review and seen again six months later when apart from some dental fricative fronting, which was appropriate at her age, all simplifying processes were resolved. It is possible that Ruth's relatively straightforward problems would have resolved spontaneously over time. Nevertheless we feel that the decision to provide therapy was an appropriate one. A small amount of therapy, approximately eight hours in total, led to quick resolution of all her simplifying processes.

Example 3

Will was 3;8 at the start of therapy. He was the younger of two children. Developmental milestones were normal and there was no significant medical history. His language comprehension, as measured by the RDLS, was slightly below average and he had an age appropriate score on the BPVS. There is a family history of speech and language problems.

The following simplifying processes had a greater than 50% occurrence in his speech:

Stopping of affricates	syllable initial
Final consonant deletion	stops and approximants
Final consonant deletion	fricatives and affricates
Initial consonant cluster reduction	fricative + consonant
Initial consonant cluster reduction	plosive + consonant
Final consonant cluster deletion	

This phonological profile is notable for the preponderance of structural processes with only one systemic process, stopping of affricates. Will's phonetic inventory showed that he had all sounds in his system except affricates, but his scores on the imitation task were very poor.

This child was regarded as a suitable candidate for therapy in view of the family history of speech and language problems, the nature of the simplifying processes, and his age appropriate consonant inventory, which he was not fully exploiting.

It was decided to target the final consonant deletion process first followed by stopping of affricates. Whilst the latter is not an early resolving process, it was the only class of sounds that Will did not possess.

Will had nine sessions of therapy for final consonant deletion but they had little effect on process occurrence. This was followed by nine sessions working on stopping of affricates. Some progress was made in changing both these processes but it was rather limited and there was little generalisation to connected speech. Further therapy was required. This was provided by another therapist and we have been unable to find out about subsequent progress. We expected Metaphon therapy to have a better outcome for this child. His inventory showed that he had most phonemes in his system and during therapy sessions was able to produce affricates and on occasions make corrections in response to listener misunderstanding. The case notes suggest that Will was an unreflective child who was not very interested in the therapy activities. This may be part of the explanation but the notes also show that were frequent and often long gaps between therapy sessions for various reasons. Metaphon was probably an appropriate strategy for Will but our lack of success in getting him fully involved in therapy tasks, compounded by his poor attendance record, was responsible for the rather disappointing result in his case.

Example 4

Mike was 4;5 at the start of therapy. He was the younger of two children. His developmental milestones were normal but he had a history of persistent recurrent upper respiratory tract infections. His scores on both the BPVS and the RDLS were slightly below normal.

Mike was using the following simplifying processes at a greater than 50% occurrence at the start of therapy:

Velar fronting	syllable initial and final
Stopping of fricatives	syllable initial and final
Stopping of affricates	syllable initial and final
Liquid/glide simplification	syllable initial
Syllable initial voicing	plosives
Initial consonant cluster reduction	plosive + consonant.
Initial consonant cluster reduction	fricative + consonant.

A marked feature of Mike's phonological profile was the predominance of stopping in the systemic processes. His consonant inventory showed that fricatives were restricted to /s;z/ and /θ/ and he had no affricates. His imitative ability tended to be rather poor.

At the age of 4;5, with this range of simplifying processes, he was an obvious candidate for therapy.

The decision on what process to target first was relatively easy in this case. We decided to target stopping of fricatives first. Mike had 12 sessions (6 hours) working on this process. This led to some reduction in percentage occurrence of this process but progress was slow and there was no initial evidence of any generalisation. We then moved on to target liquid glide simplification as it was thought that working on a very different process would provide time to allow for the possibility of generalisation. This process was targeted for 10 sessions (5 hours) and once again although progress was made the process was not entirely eliminated.

Mike was put on review and seen again six months later. At this time there was marked phonological change and considerable generalisation had taken place. He maintained adult contrasts between all phonemes in all word positions in the phonological assessment. There was the occasional error in connected speech but he was consistently intelligible. No further therapy was thought necessary. This considerable change after therapy was discontinued is very interesting given the rather slow progress he made during treatment, which was rather longer than average for both processes.

The case notes provide relevant clues to Mike's pattern of change. He was a child who, initially, was very passive during therapy. Throughout the whole period of his therapy he would work hard on tasks that interested him but refuse to co-operate if they did not. He appeared unreflective during Phase 1 activities but a marked change was noted after Phase 2 activities were introduced. He then became very responsive to listener uncertainty and was heard to comment on his own pronunciation. The therapist noted throughout her evaluation of therapy sessions with Mike that he became particularly uncooperative if he sensed that pressure was being put upon him to produce sounds. He was particularly reluctant to attempt fricatives which suggests that although he was aware of what was required he lacked the appropriate knowledge, or ability, to make the required changes. She also reported that he seemed to have difficulty in producing /r/ when working on liquid glide simplification.

It is possible that the most important factor in bringing about the alteration in Mike's system was the realisation that he would need to make changes if he was to be understood. His apparent lack of enjoyment of some of the Phase 1 tasks is unusual and there are two possible explanations for this. It perhaps resulted from some actual, or presumed, difficulty on his part with producing speech sounds. If this was the case, Phase 2 activities may have helped him to overcome this, resulting in slow but ultimately successful phonological change. It could be argued that therapy focusing directly on articulatory placement might have been more successful but, given Mike's reluctance to co-operate in activities connected with producing sounds, it is difficult to see how he could have been persuaded to take part in such therapy. Alternatively it is possible that his lack of enjoyment resulted from poor reflective skills or metaphonological constraints which were modified as a result of therapy. If this was the case he might have benefited from participation in a group which provided the opportunity for him to enhance his reflective ability and general language awareness before being given a course of individual Metaphon therapy. To conclude, it will never be possible to determine whether the marked change in Mike's speech after therapy had stopped was part of a continuing change that had been instigated during intervention, or was the result of maturation. We believe that Metaphon was an appropriate therapy for Mike but his response raises questions about ways in which this approach might be modified to suit the specific needs of individual children, a point we take up again in Chapter 9.

We will now look at the data from three more of our phonologically disordered children. For these children we will start our discussion at the stage at which the simplifying processes were revealed by their screening assessments so that we can say what Process Specific Probes were applied, chart the outcome of this procedure and say what resulting treatment decisions were made. We will also refer briefly to the outcome of treatment. The treatment activities for each of these three children is discussed in more detail in Chapter 7. For ease of comparison we will use the same descriptive format for each child.

Example 5

Jack was an only child and he was 3;8 at the start of therapy. Language development was reported as being very delayed but other developmental milestones were normal and there was no significant medical history. His score on the RDLS was above average, but he had slightly below average vocabulary as measured by the BPVS.

Administration of the MRP Screening Procedure showed that the following processes were operating in Jack's speech:

Systemic processes

Velar fronting
Palato-alveolar fronting
Stopping of fricatives
Stopping of affricates
Syllable initial voicing
Liquid gliding
Dental Fronting

Structural processes

Initial consonant deletion
Initial cluster reduction

We will discuss each of the processes listed above in turn, say whether we decided to probe the process, give the results of the probes and say whether they should be targeted in therapy.

Velar Fronting

This occurred in one of the four word initial screening examples and two of the four word final screening examples. A Process Specific Probe was applied to enable us to look, particularly, at word final occurrence in more detail. This probe confirmed the general pattern of occurrence found in screening that this process occurred only once word initially and medially but in 63% of word final contexts. Figure 5 provides a summary of percentage occurrence of all the processes we probed.

Occurrence of velar fronting (word finally) did not appear to be restricted to specific phonemes; some but not all voiced and voiceless stops and nasals were fronted. Because this pattern of selective operation suggested that Jack may have been spontaneously eliminating this

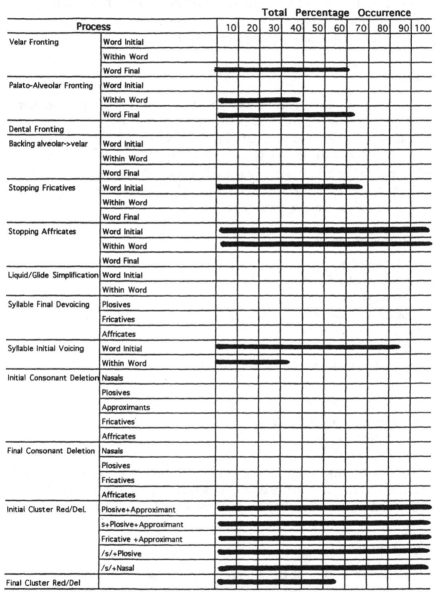

Figure 5 Percentage occurrence simplifying phonological processes, Process Specific Probes (Jack, chronological age 3;8)

process from his speech it was not considered as an initial candidate for treatment. As this process is not recorded in the normal development stages after the age of 2;6 (Grunwell, 1985) it was reviewed later to see if spontaneous elimination had occurred.

Palato-alveolar Fronting

In the screening data for palato-alveolar fronting, the same pattern of predominance in word final position occurred that was evident in velar fronting. But it was noted that Jack did not use the adult target word initially, but instead of fronting used another simplifying process, stopping. A Process Specific Probe confirmed this pattern of distribution.

Again it appears that spontaneous resolution may have been taking place. This process still occurs in normally developing speech between the ages of 3 and 3;6. Because of both these factors it was not considered to require treatment but again review was advisable.

Stopping of Fricatives

This occurred in more than 50% of word initial contexts, but not word final contexts in the screening data. A Process Specific Probe was carried out which confirmed occurrence word initially, at 65%, but no word medial or word final occurrence (Figure 5). Further examination of the probe data showed that the stopping process was applied to /s; z; θ; ð/) but /f/ and /v/ were both realised as [w], that is they were subject to a different simplifying process.

Although stopping of some fricatives is still recorded in normal development up to the age of 3;6, notably of /v/ and /z/, the consistency of the application of this process to certain phonemes word initially suggested that this was a suitable process for treatment.

Stopping of Affricates

This occurred in 100% of word initial situations in the screening procedure, but not word finally. A Process Specific Probe confirmed 100% occurrence both word initially and within word (see Figure 5), but Jack did use affricates in most word final positions.

Stopping of affricates will tend to resolve later than stopping of fricatives. This process was therefore reviewed after treatment for stopping of fricatives to determine whether it had resolved.

Syllable Initial Voicing

The screening procedure showed this was a frequently occurring process and a Process Specific Probe was therefore carried out. Figure

5 shows that the process occurred in 83% of word initial and 33% of word within contexts. Examination of the data sample also showed that fricatives which were subject to the stopping process were also voiced, for example /s/ was realised as [d] so 'sun' became [dʌn].

Syllable initial voicing was therefore predominant in this child's speech and as it is not reported after the age of three in normal development (Grunwell, 1985) it was a suitable candidate for therapy.

Liquid Glide Simplification

This process was only noted in one of the four possible screening occurrences. It was therefore not investigated further.

Dental Fronting

This process did not occur word initially but in 100% of word final positions in the screening procedure. As this process is reported as occurring in normal children up to the age of 4;6 and above, it did not require further investigation at this stage.

Initial Consonant Deletion

This was only recorded in one out of six possible occurrences in the screening procedure and was therefore not investigated further.

Initial Cluster Reduction

There was 100% occurrence of this process in the screening assessment. A Process Specific Probe confirmed that Jack reduced all word initial clusters to one element. Normally developing children may reduce all clusters up to the age of 3 but would have started to use a range of stop+approximant and /s/+consonant clusters by Jack's age, 3;8. Initial cluster reduction was therefore considered as a target for therapy.

Final Cluster Reduction

Two out of the three screening occurrences of this process were reduced to one element. Application of a Process Specific Probe confirmed this picture with a 55% occurrence. Further scrutiny of the data showed nasal+stop clusters to be well established word finally. Further review was to be carried out after providing treatment for initial cluster reduction.

Figure 6 shows Jack's consonant inventory. It was considered to be almost age appropriate. He used all fricatives except /θ;ð;ʒ/ and showed no use of affricate /tʃ/.

	LABIAL		DENTAL		ALVEOLAR		POST-ALVEOLAR		PALATAL	VELAR		GLOTTAL
NASAL		ⓜ				ⓝ					ⓝ(ŋ)	
PLOSIVE	p	ⓑ			ⓣ	ⓓ				k	ⓖ	
FRICATIVE	f	ⓥ	θ	ð	ⓢ	ⓩ	ⓕ(ʃ)	ʒ		x		ⓗ
AFFRICATE							tʃ	ⓓʒ				
APPROXIMANT	ʍ	ⓦ				ⓛ		ɹ	j			
TRILL						r						

Figure 6 Consonant inventory (Jack, chronological age 3;8)

Summary

We have considered each process separately and have made some reference to the age at which processes spontaneously resolve and given some indication as to whether they were possible targets for therapy. We now need to consider the overall picture of this child and discuss the order in which processes were treated. Before doing this we did of course make a decision about whether treatment was required at all or whether some other management strategy should be adopted.

In making a decision about whether to provide treatment in this case we took the following factors into consideration. Firstly age: Jack was very young, only 3;8. He was, however, advanced for his age in other aspects of language development and general cognitive functioning. He was also becoming frustrated when he was not understood.

If we consider the nature of the processes that were operating in Jack's speech, we find that these were overwhelmingly developmental in nature and apart from cluster reduction were optional in application. Examination of his consonant system (Figure 6) shows that Jack could make most of the sounds that he was not using appropriately to signal contrasts.

If we look only at Jack's speech characteristics, these factors suggest that phonological development may proceed relatively quickly without intervention. However, because of Jack's frustration and his advanced ability in other language skills we decided to provide him with a course of treatment.

A decision then had to be made about which processes to target first. On the basis of the Process Specific Probe results the prime candidates were considered to be syllable initial voicing, stopping of fricatives, velar fronting and initial cluster reduction.

Velar fronting appeared to show most evidence of spontaneous resolution. Therefore it was not chosen as an initial target for therapy in the hope that it might resolve spontaneously. Treatment of initial cluster reduction was not appropriate until both syllable initial voicing and stopping of fricatives, which were both prevalent word initially, were resolved. The full range of reduced clusters could then be worked on together.

It was decided to work on syllable initial voicing first followed by stopping of fricatives, primarily because some fricatives which were stopped were also voiced. If syllable initial voicing was eliminated first, all stopped fricatives could then be remediated together. A different decision may be taken for other children where both these processes are operating if the pattern of application is different, particularly as both processes disappear developmentally at approximately the same time.

Outcome

In the event this appeared to be an appropriate choice of targets. Jack received a total of 14 thirty-minute treatment sessions over a period of six months (details of this treatment can be found in Chapter 7). Approximately half of the treatment sessions were targeted at syllable initial voicing and half at stopping of fricatives.

Review at the end of the treatment period showed that both treated processes had completely disappeared. In addition spontaneous resolution of cluster reduction was also occurring, and velar fronting had resolved although there was still some evidence of palato-alveolar fronting and liquid gliding. It was decided that no further treatment was required at this stage, and when reviewed again six months later, that is one year after first starting treatment, Jack had no simplifying processes except dental fronting; he was therefore discharged.

Example 6

Barry was 4;3 at the start of therapy. He was the younger of two children. Language was reported as being delayed until the age of two but then developed rapidly. Developmental milestones were normal and there was no significant medical history. He had an average score on the RDLS and a slightly above average score on the BPVS.

The screening assessment revealed the presence of the following processes:

Systemic processes

Velar fronting
Stopping of fricatives
Stopping of affricates
Syllable initial voicing

Structural processes

Initial consonant deletion
Initial cluster reduction

We will discuss each of the processes listed above in turn, say whether we decided to probe the process, give the results of the probes and say whether they should be targeted in therapy.

Velar Fronting

This occurred in all word initial items in the screening procedure. A Process Specific Probe was therefore carried out. As Figure 7 shows, this confirmed the results of the screening procedure; there was 100% occurrence of this process word initially but it did not occur word medially or finally.

Though the operation of this process was confined to word initial position, its obligatory use in this context suggested that it was a suitable process for treatment. Note that, for Barry, unlike Jack, velar fronting was not accompanied by palato-alveolar fronting. This was not because Barry used the adult target for these sounds but because they were subject to other processes as we shall see below.

Stopping of Fricatives

In the screening procedure all fricatives were stopped within words and in all word final positions, but not word initially. The Process Specific Probe showed that there was 100% occurrence of this process word medially and finally (Figure 7). This process did not operate word initially because all fricatives were omitted in this position, as we shall see below. This illustrates the complex inter-relationship between the operation of processes that we referred to earlier in this chapter. Stopping of fricatives would appear to be a candidate for treatment.

Stopping of Affricates

The Process Specific Probe showed that this process was operating at 100% occurrence word initially and finally and 50% occurrence within words. It is interesting to note that in word initial position Barry did not treat affricates in the same way as fricatives, by omitting them, but used instead the stop element of the phoneme. We therefore get 'cheep' as [tip] but 'sharp' as [ap].

This process would be reviewed again after treatment for stopping of fricatives, and then treated if required.

Process		Total Percentage Occurrence									
		10	20	30	40	50	60	70	80	90	100
Velar Fronting	Word Initial	▬	▬	▬	▬	▬	▬	▬	▬	▬	▬
	Within Word										
	Word Final										
Palato-Alveolar Fronting	Word Initial										
	Within Word										
	Word Final										
Dental Fronting											
Backing alveolar->velar	Word Initial										
	Within Word										
	Word Final										
Stopping Fricatives	Word Initial										
	Within Word	▬	▬	▬	▬	▬	▬	▬	▬	▬	▬
	Word Final	▬	▬	▬	▬	▬	▬	▬	▬	▬	▬
Stopping Affricates	Word Initial	▬	▬	▬	▬	▬	▬	▬	▬	▬	▬
	Within Word	▬	▬	▬	▬	▬					
	Word Final	▬	▬	▬	▬	▬	▬	▬	▬	▬	▬
Liquid/Glide Simplification	Word Initial										
	Within Word										
Syllable Final Devoicing	Plosives										
	Fricatives										
	Affricates										
Syllable Initial Voicing	Word Initial										
	Within Word										
Initial Consonant Deletion	Nasals										
	Plosives										
	Approximants	▬	▬	▬	▬						
	Fricatives	▬	▬	▬	▬	▬	▬	▬	▬	▬	▬
	Affricates										
Final Consonant Deletion	Nasals										
	Plosives										
	Fricatives										
	Affricates										
Initial Cluster Red/Del.	Plosive+Approximant	▬	▬	▬	▬	▬	▬	▬	▬	▬	▬
	s+Plosive+Approximant	▬	▬	▬	▬	▬	▬	▬	▬	▬	▬
	Fricative +Approximant	▬	▬	▬	▬	▬	▬	▬	▬	▬	▬
	/s/+Plosive	▬	▬	▬	▬	▬	▬	▬	▬	▬	▬
	/s/+Nasal	▬	▬	▬	▬	▬	▬	▬	▬	▬	▬
Final Cluster Red/Del											

Key: Red/Del = Reduction / Deletion

Figure 7 Percentage occurrence simplifying phonological processes, Process Specific Probes (Barry, chronological age 4;3)

Syllable Initial Voicing

This occurred in seven of the possible screening items, but it did not appear to be consistently applied to any particular phonemes or sound classes. It did not therefore need further investigation at that time.

Initial Consonant Deletion

An examination of the screening transcript showed this to be a particularly prevalent process. It was therefore investigated further with a Process Specific Probe. Figure 7 reveals the following pattern of distribution: no nasals or stops were deleted, but there was 100% deletion of fricatives. Approximant /r/ was also deleted, but other approximants were used word initially and, as we saw above, affricates were realised as stops. This process is perhaps therefore more accurately described as 'initial *fricative* deletion'.

This is an atypical process and contributed considerably to Barry's unintelligibility; it was therefore considered as an urgent candidate for treatment.

Initial Cluster Reduction and Deletion

It is not surprising to find that the screening procedure revealed 100% cluster reduction. The Process Specific Probe showed the same pattern. Closer inspection of the data showed that Barry reduced rather than deleted clusters, with the exception of some deletion of fricative+ approximant clusters, for example 'three' as [i]. These patterns of reduction and deletion were consistent with the pattern of the operation of initial consonant deletion.

As Figure 8 shows, Barry had a very reduced consonant system. He had no fricatives or affricates in his system. It is not difficult to imagine therefore that he experienced considerable difficulty in making himself understood. An interesting phonetic feature was the production of /s/ as [tʰtʰ] word finally so that grass was realised as [datʰtʰ]. This realisation can be interpreted as possible evidence that Barry had some concept of length or frication that he was attempting to represent.

Summary

Phonological analysis left us in no doubt that Barry required treatment. He presented with a variety of simplifying processes including an atypical process of initial consonant deletion.

	LABIAL		DENTAL		ALVEOLAR		POST-ALVEOLAR	PALATAL	VELAR		GLOTTAL
NASAL		(m)				(n)				(ŋ)	
PLOSIVE	(p)	(b)			(t)	(d)			(k)	(g)	
FRICATIVE	f	v	θ	ð	s	z	ʃ 3		x		h
AFFRICATE							ʧ dʒ				
APPROXIMANT	ʍ	(w)				(ɹ)		(j)			
TRILL					r						

Figure 8 Consonant inventory (Barry, chronological age 4;3)

In making decisions about where to start treatment we gave some consideration to his consonant inventory. We can see from Figure 8 that his problems could in part be accounted for by the absence of any fricatives in his inventory. However, as we saw earlier, the use of [tʰtʰ] word finally provides a possible indication that Barry had some concept of length or frication which he was attempting to represent.

Velar fronting, stopping of fricatives, initial fricative deletion and cluster reduction all required attention. It was decided to treat velar fronting first on the basis that generalisation of phonemes that were already in his system to all word positions would provide a motivating start to treatment. Initial fricative deletion was treated next on the grounds that the introduction of fricatives word initially might lead automatically to the elimination of stopping in other word positions. If generalisation of frication did not occur treatment would be provided for this process, followed by treatment for cluster reduction if this did not resolve spontaneously.

Outcome

Barry received seven half hour treatment sessions for velar fronting followed by 13 sessions for initial fricative deletion over a period of six months (see Chapter 7 for details of therapy activities and response to therapy). Reassessment at this time showed that both treated processes had completely resolved. Stopping of fricatives and stopping of affricates were still present but confined to word final position. There was some liquid gliding whilst cluster reduction was starting to resolve spontaneously and was restricted to stops+approximants and /s/+stop+approximants. Therapy was therefore continued for another two months, during which time treatment was provided for stopping of fricatives and liquid gliding. When Barry's progress was reviewed after a further three months, that is one year after the start of therapy, all processes had resolved and there was no need for further treatment.

Example 7

Jamie was 4;7 at the start of therapy. He was the younger of two children. Language was reported as being slightly slow to develop but other developmental milestones were normal. There was no significant medical history. His standard score on the RDLS was well above average and average on the BPVS.

The screening assessment showed that the following processes were operating in Jamie's speech.

Systemic processes

Velar fronting
Palato-alveolar fronting of fricatives

Other processes were also operating (see below).

Stopping of affricates
Backing of alveolar stops
Syllable initial voicing
Liquid gliding
Dental Fronting

Structural processes

Initial consonant deletion
Initial cluster reduction and deletion

As with the other two children we will look at each of these processes in turn. The pattern of simplifying processes operating in Jamie's speech revealed by more detailed examination was as follows.

Velar Fronting

This process was confined to velar nasal /ŋ/ which was optionally fronted to [n] word finally. This was not considered to be a major problem and no further investigation was undertaken.

Palato-alveolar Fronting

Fricatives /s; z; ʃ; ʒ / were realised as [f; v] within word and word finally. This appeared to be an obligatory process in word final positions so a Process Specific Probe was administered. The probe (Figure 9) showed a 100% occurrence within words and 78% occurrence word finally. This process was not operating word initially because palato-alveolar sounds were omitted or stopped in this position. The operation of these processes will be discussed below. Palato-alveolar fronting of this kind was regarded as a candidate for treatment.

Backing Alveolar Stops

This occurred in more than 50% of the possible occurrences in the screening procedure so a Process Specific Probe was undertaken. The probe revealed that this process was operating 50% word initially and 100% within words and word finally (Figure 9). More detailed investigation showed that word initially backing was confined to voiced stops; voiceless stops were omitted in this position. Backing is an atypical process and it required treatment.

Syllable Initial Voicing

Although this process occurred in less than 50% of those items used in the screening procedure, examination of the data collection sheet

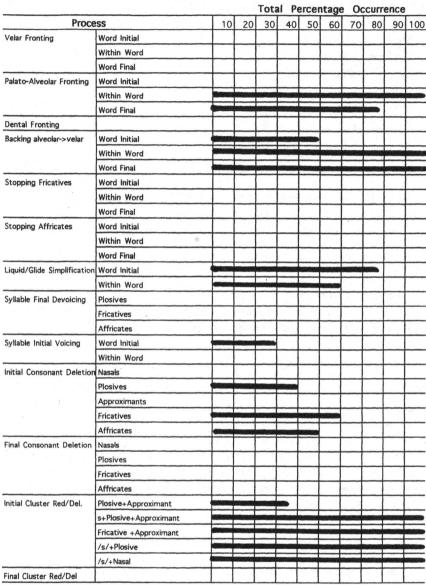

Figure 9 Percentage occurrence simplifying phonological processes, Process Specific Probes (Jamie, chronological age 4;7)

showed that stop elements of clusters were also frequently voiced and that word final voiceless stops were sometimes voiced. A Process Specific Probe was therefore administered. The probe showed that /p/ word initially was always voiced and realised as [b]. Alveolar and velar voiceless stops /t/ and /k/ were subject to another process, initial consonant deletion. It was concluded that syllable initial voicing required treatment at some stage.

Liquid Gliding

This occurred in 50% of possible screening items. The Process Specific Probe showed that there was a 78% occurrence of this process word initially and a 60% occurrence within words. More detailed examination showed that this process could be accounted for entirely by the realisation of /l/ and /r/ as [w]. This process is reported to be used by some normal children up to the age of 4;6. It was not therefore considered to require treatment at this stage but should be re-assessed later.

Initial Consonant Deletion

The screening transcript showed consistent deletion of some stops and fricatives word initially so a Process Specific Probe was administered. The probe revealed that all voiceless fricatives and affricates and all voiceless alveolar and velar stops were deleted word initially. The consequent relative percentage occurrence can be found in Figure 9. This is another atypical process that required treatment.

Initial Cluster Reduction and Deletion

The screening assessment showed this to be a prominent process and this was confirmed by the Process Specific Probe. There was 100% reduction or deletion of all initial clusters with the exception of stop+approximants which showed 35% occurrence (see Figure 9). This process may be a candidate for treatment at a later stage in the therapy programme if reassessment does not show spontaneous change.

Other Processes

In addition to the processes listed above which are specifically investigated by the MRP some other processes were observed to occur in Jamie's speech. These appeared, for the most part, to be in accord with the general pattern of the processes listed above. They included backing of /ʤ/ to [g] and some instances of /n/ to [ŋ], voicing of some word final voiceless stops and realisation of /s/ and /ʃ / as [f] and [v].

Figure 10 shows that Jamie had a very restricted consonant inventory for his age (4;7). Fricatives were restricted to /f/,/v/ and a bi-labial voiceless fricative /ɸ/ which does not occur in English. Jamie had no alveolar stops and the alveolar place of articulation was represented only by /n/ and /l/.

Summary

There were numerous processes operating in Jamie's speech, some of them being atypical and at the age of 4;7 he clearly required therapy. This example shows that although Jamie had a complex set of processes they did conform to a systematic pattern. The data sample showed for example that he deleted all classes of voiceless phonemes word initially and tended to back voiced phonemes from the same classes.

	LABIAL		DENTAL		ALVEOLAR		POST-ALVEOLAR	PALATAL	VELAR		GLOTTAL
NASAL		m				n				ŋ	
PLOSIVE	p	b			t	d			k	g	
FRICATIVE	f ɸ	v	θ	ð	s	z	ʃ	ʒ	x		h
AFFRICATE							ʧ	ʤ			
APPROXIMANT	ʍ	w				l		j	l		
TRILL						r					

Figure 10 Consonant inventory (Jamie, chronological age 4;7)

Discovering patterns such as this in the child's pronunciation is essential if specifically targeted therapy is to be provided. These patterns will not be revealed, however, without close examination of the data.

We have used Jamie's data as an example because it illustrates very vividly the complexity of some children's problems but it also shows that this complexity can be disentangled with probing analysis, which can then be followed by appropriate treatment. Comparison of Jamie's consonant inventory (Figure 10), which had few fricatives, and very restricted use of the alveolar place of articulation, was reflected in the processes that were operating in his speech.

We have seen that there were several processes that required treatment. The most urgent appeared to be initial consonant deletion and backing. A decision was made to treat initial consonant deletion first because, it was argued, we could in this way maximise the use of phonemes Jamie was already using and possibly encourage the production and use of alveolar sounds across different classes for use in word initial position. This would be followed by work to eliminate backing, once again reinforcing the production and use of the alveolar place of articulation across all classes of sounds. Such a treatment regime, working as it does across a variety of sounds, is economical in treatment time and should also result in a rapid increase in intelligibility.

Liquid gliding, palato-alveolar fronting, syllable initial voicing and cluster reduction also required attention, but decisions would be made about the order of treatment for these remaining processes after the effects of treatment on initial consonant deletion and backing had been reviewed.

Outcome

Unfortunately this child moved out of our district so we are not able to comment on the final outcome of treatment. He received 13 sessions of Metaphon therapy over a period of three months. Treatment was given for initial consonant deletion and backing (see Chapter 7 for more information).

On reassessment at the end of this time initial consonant deletion had been completely eliminated and backing had decreased. There was some spontaneous resolution of syllable initial voicing, liquid gliding and palato-alveolar fronting and cluster reduction was confined to /s/+stop and /s/+stop+approximant.

An outstanding feature of Jamie's reaction to treatment was his ability to self monitor and spontaneously correct any errors he made. We have every confidence that this ability and the rapid improvement he made during his time with us should have ensured that he acquired normal pronunciation patterns within a relatively short time.

Conclusion

We can now summarise our discussion of the speech patterns of these three children. We have discussed them in order of severity. Although they presented with different problems they had processes in common. For instance all made extensive use of initial cluster reduction, two used stopping of fricatives and all three used syllable initial voicing. They all displayed different patterns of use of these processes, however, in that they each used them differently in different word positions and to different extents.

Barry and Jamie had the most severe problems. They both used an atypical process of initial consonant deletion and Jamie who had the most complex disordered system also made extensive use of another atypical process, backing. Both these children, unlike Jack, had restricted consonant inventories which can be seen, at least in part, to be responsible for the simplifying processes. Barry's inventory was notable for its lack of fricatives and Jamie's for its reduced fricative system and a reluctance to use alveolar place of articulation.

It is important to point out that in neither case could these reduced consonant inventories be accounted for by articulatory difficulties. Both children had no difficulty in imitating the consonants that were not in their systems and they were able to use all these missing sounds freely in therapeutic activities from the start of treatment. At no time was either child given any phonetic exercises or specific instruction on how to make these consonants.

We hope the inclusion of this data from these seven children helps to illuminate the nature of phonological disorder and demonstrate how information about the precise nature of speech patterns determines treatment planning in Metaphon therapy. This chapter has been concerned to show that phonological analysis provides the essential basis for treatment planning. It establishes what processes require treatment and how such treatment should be ordered.

Having established what requires treatment the next two chapters will discuss the theory which underlies Metaphon therapy.

Chapter 4
Theoretical Basis:
Metalinguistic Ability

In this the first of our two chapters concerned with the theoretical basis of Metaphon we examine what we believe phonologically disordered children need to learn in the therapeutic situation to help them make the phonological changes they require. In the next chapter we discuss ways in which the optimum conditions for this learning can be provided.

The fundamental purpose of remediation for these children must be to ensure that they reach the same level of phonological development as other children of their age and psycholinguistic ability. Our methods for achieving this purpose arise directly from our belief that their difficulties lie primarily in their failure to acquire the adult rules of their native language rather than with producing speech sounds. Our aim therefore is to give these children the ability to acquire and apply the adult rules in their speech output.

But how can we achieve this aim? It is not possible to directly access and change the processes that are going on in the children's heads to effect change in their speech. When children have problems with physically articulating sounds we may, for instance, show them where to put the tongue to produce a more acceptable sound. Such instruction is not appropriate or helpful for children who have phonological difficulties. Similarly, providing target words for the child to imitate, even if the targets are contrastive minimal pairs, will be of limited value because, as we demonstrated earlier, these children are not fully aware of the nature of their communication failure. They may sense in some way that they have problems in communicating with others, but the very nature of their problem indicates that they have little knowledge of the precise nature of their difficulty.

We would argue that the most satisfactory way of helping these children to change their rule systems and consequent speech output is to provide them with information which will encourage them to make their own changes. We believe that they will be unable to review and revise their existing rule system, and consequent speech output, unless the following conditions, which we referred to in Chapter 2, can be met:

1. Knowledge that change is required.
2. Knowledge that change can be made.
3. Information about how that change might be achieved.
(See also Hewlett, 1990; Howell and McCartney, 1990.)

Metaphon attempts to fulfil these conditions through a series of activities aimed at increasing children's knowledge of language and encouraging them to reflect about the nature of language. That is, in Metaphon therapy we have attempted to overcome the children's disabilities by developing and utilising their metalinguistic ability.

We can summarise our approach by saying that we have adopted an alternative perspective to intervention for these children. We do not concentrate primarily on 'on-line' linguistic processing (input, decoding, encoding, realisation) and attempt to overcome particular weaknesses along this continuum, the conventional treatment approach for this population. Instead the basic focus of Metaphon therapy is on the children's cognitive abilities and the development of knowledge that they can use to facilitate change in their speech output. We would not, however, ignore the need to search for potential individual weaknesses; we argued in Chapter 2 for the importance of comprehensive assessment. If such assessment reveals any specific processing limitations Metaphon therapy can be adapted to compensate for these. We discuss some of the ways this can be done in Chapter 9.

In this chapter we will look first at the concept of metalinguistic ability. We will then outline how we utilise aspects of linguistic awareness in Metaphon and accompany this with some examples of similar sorts of activities that have been observed in normal development. After this we will examine theories that postulate a possible role for awareness in phonological development, and we will end the chapter by discussing the metalinguistic abilities of language disordered children. Several of the points we make in this chapter will be taken up again in more detail when we discuss how children learn in Chapter 5 and in Chapter 6 where we give a detailed description of Metaphon therapy.

The Concept of Metalinguistic Ability

Metalinguistic ability has been described by Cazden (1972: p. 303) as 'The ability to reflect upon language as well as comprehend and produce it' and by Pratt and Grieve (1984a: p.2) as 'The ability to think about and reflect upon the nature and functions of language'. In essence when we are talking about linguistic awareness we are concerned with the ability to consider language, or an aspect of language, as a tangible entity, an object in itself separated from its meaning. In

Metaphon therapy we are particularly concerned with utilising and developing phonological awareness but it should be noted that it is possible to reflect upon any aspect of language. For instance we can give our attention to the grammatical structure of language, the meanings of words and the way that we use language to communicate.

The nature of metalinguistic ability is such that it is not a clearly defined, universally agreed concept. The boundaries between using and reflecting upon language are not clearly drawn and there is controversy about the age at which children are said to be able to demonstrate awareness of language and indeed what constitutes evidence of awareness. It is not appropriate to enter into detailed discussion about the theoretical arguments surrounding the concept of metalinguistic ability in this volume except to say a little more about the age at which children are said to be able to reflect upon language. There are three main viewpoints:

1. Awareness develops alongside language itself. It is argued that as the child's language grows and develops so does the ability to reflect more deeply about more aspects of language.
2. It is an ability that develops in middle childhood and is related to the more general development of information processing capability which occurs during this period.
3. It develops around the start of formal schooling and is associated with learning to read.

Further information and critical evaluation of the concept of linguistic awareness can be found in Sinclair, Jarvella and Levelt (1978), Tunmer and Herriman (1984), Garton and Pratt (1989) and Gombert (1992).

The first view listed above, that metalinguistic ability develops alongside language, is the one that is of direct relevance to Metaphon therapy. There is a considerable amount of observational evidence to support this viewpoint.

The main source of this evidence comes from descriptions of children playing with and manipulating the phonological structure of language and making spontaneous repairs (corrections) to their utterances if they are not understood (we will provide some examples of these activities later in the chapter). This type of behaviour has been reported in children aged from about 18 months or so. Such observations suggest that children from this very young age know something about, at least, some aspects of language, in particular its phonemic composition.

Understandably, it is difficult to obtain experimental evidence of explicit reflection about language at this very young age, but some investigators have successfully elicited explicit judgements about syntax and semantics from two and three year old children by asking them if sentences they were asked to listen to sounded 'good' or 'silly' (de Villiers and de Villiers, 1972; Gleitman, Gleitman and Shipley, 1972).

Awareness of phonological structure is usually determined experimentally by assessing recognition or generation of rhyming words or ability to segment words into their constituent phonemes. Attempts to elicit explicit phonemic awareness by these methods from pre-school children initially met with little success. Early investigators tended to conclude that children showed little awareness of this aspect of language until after they had started school at the age of five or six. Examination of this research suggests that the explanation for this apparent lack of phonemic awareness may rest partly on the metalinguistic requirements of the tasks used in some of the experiments and partly on the way in which these tasks were designed and presented.

There is strong evidence to suggest a developmental progression in phonemic awareness. Rhyme recognition is easier than segmentation and different types of segmentation activities appear to present with different degrees of difficulty. Both rhyming and segmentation require auditory perceptual ability and some appreciation of the phonemic composition of words. But rhyming tasks, although they require the knowledge that words share common phonemes that can be matched and categorised, do not require the ability to detach these phonemes from other phonemes in the word. This ability is required, however, for success in segmentation tasks where specific characteristics of a phoneme, usually the initial phoneme, have to be determined and extracted from the co-occurring acoustic characteristics of other phonemes in the word.

Recent investigations, for example Chaney (1992) and Reid et al. (1993), have shown that some pre-school children can successfully participate in phonemic awareness experiments if the experimental tasks are carefully designed on the basis of metalinguistic task requirements and take into account memory and other cognitive limitations of this age group.

We will describe the metalinguistic research undertaken by ourselves and our colleagues (Reid et al., 1993) to provide an example of the sort of experiments that can be used to elicit metalinguistic judgements in pre-school children. These experiments form part of the second Metaphon efficacy study, more information about which can be found in Chapter 8.

We devised three metalinguistic tasks for the study, two tests of phonological awareness – rhyme awareness and phoneme awareness, and a word order task. The tasks were carefully designed so that they captured the children's interest. We also tried to minimise cognitive demands which might interfere with the children's ability to exercise their metalinguistic abilities, by using short instructions, a minimum of metalinguistic terminology and clear demonstration and practice items.

As we were going to use the tasks with phonologically disordered, as well as normally developing children, they were designed so that only non-verbal or minimal verbal responses were required. Because the tasks were part of a larger battery of tests that were being administered by speech and language therapists participating in the efficacy project we also made sure that each task took no more than ten minutes to administer. In order to maintain reliability across this large group of testers we also tried to ensure that the tests were straightforward to administer and score.

In the word order task the children are shown a toy parrot that they are told is learning to talk. The children are asked to help the parrot by judging whether the 'stories' (sentences) it tells are 'good' or 'mixed up'. The 20 test items were assembled from 10 semantically similar sentence pairs, such as 'wash your face' and 'dry your hands'. For each pair one sentence was allocated randomly to the correct word order condition (e.g. 'wash your face') and the other to the reverse order condition (e.g. 'hands your dry').

The rhyme awareness task was adapted from Read (1978). In this task the children were asked whether words rhymed with the name of a puppet called 'Ed'. In our investigation the children are introduced to the task through nursery rhymes. 'Ed' is a toy monkey and the children are asked to decide whether he would like certain words. Twenty items are used, five rhyming words , five rhyming non-words , five non-rhyming words and five non-rhyming non-words. For example 'red', 'med', 'house' and 'bouse' respectively.

In the phoneme awareness task the children are asked to detect a word initial target phoneme, given a choice of three monosyllabic words which differ only in their initial consonant, for example 'pear', 'hair' and 'bear'. To minimise memory load each set of words is accompanied by amusing cartoon drawings like the example in Figure 11.

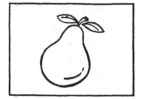 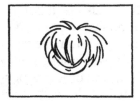 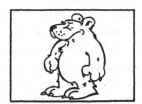

Figure 11 Phoneme awareness task items (from Reid et al., 1993)

There are 12 sets of words in total; six sets sample the ability to detect /s/ and six /b/. These particular targets were chosen because it is suggested that some sounds are easier to detect than others. In a previous study (Reid, 1989) there was an indication that the fricative /s/ was one of the easiest sounds to segment. Plosives such as /b/ may be rather more difficult to detect because they are more highly encoded in the acoustic signal than fricatives.

These awareness tasks will eventually be administered to 80 normally developing children between 3;6 and 5;5, that is, 10 children at each of eight age bands (three month intervals). There are equal numbers of girls and boys.

At the moment we have results from 55 children in the 4 to 5;5 age bands. The overall pass rate for these children, calculated on the basis of scores being significantly better than chance, was 54% on the word order task, 37% on the rhyme task and 40% on the phoneme awareness task. These results are comparable with those reported by Chaney (1992) who reports pass rates between 30% and 90% on a battery of metalinguistic tasks administered to 43 children aged between 2;9 and 4;2 (see also Vance, in press).

When we look at the relationship between task success and chronological age we find that there is a tendency for task success to increase with age in all three experiments, but this is not a clearcut increase and there is considerable overlap among the scores from the different age bands. This relationship between ability and chronological age also corresponds to results from similar investigations.

The higher pass rate for the word order task compared to the rhyme and phoneme tasks is a reflection of the relative difficulty of the latter tasks, and is in line with the results reported in previous research. Contrary to expectations, however, our children found the phoneme awareness task easier than the rhyme task. On the basis of our previous discussion of the requirements for success on these tasks we would expect the reverse to be the case. This unexpected result is perhaps a reflection of task design; the use of pictures in the phoneme task perhaps reduced memory load and/or made the task more attractive, compared to the rhyme task. It can also be argued that our task was easier than some other segmentation tasks because we gave the children specific information about the target phoneme we wished them to identify. More detailed discussion of this investigation can be found in Reid et al. (1993) and we will take up the question of syllable recognition and segmentation again in Chapter 6.

The main purpose of describing our investigation here has been to illustrate the type of tasks used to elicit linguistic awareness judgements. However, these preliminary results, which are in general agreement with those found by Chaney (1992), show that some normal pre-school children are able to demonstrate explicit phonological

awareness. Later in the chapter we will look at how phonologically disordered children compare with normally developing children on metalinguistic tasks.

Metalinguistic Ability and Metaphon

The activities we use in Metaphon therapy to facilitate phonological
change have been influenced primarily by the knowledge that children
appear to be able to focus on the phonological structure of language
and make spontaneous repairs from the age of 18 months or so. In this
section of the chapter we outline the design of Metaphon therapy,
before describing it in detail in Chapter 6, and provide some examples
of the sort of Metalinguistic activities that have been observed in young
children that are comparable to Metaphon therapy activities.

We concentrate on three aspects of linguistic awareness in
Metaphon – 'metaphonology', 'metacommunication' and 'repair strategies' – in a two phase treatment approach.

By metaphonology we mean the ability to pay attention to and
reflect upon the phonological structure of language. We help the children to realise that sounds have certain combinations of characteristics
which distinguish them from other sounds in the language but also
that some of these characteristics are shared with other sounds and as a
consequence can be grouped and categorised according to these characteristics. The first phase of Metaphon is targeted at demonstrating
these characteristics to the children and encouraging them to explore
and manipulate the sound system of their native language. In essence it
provides the third of the requirements we listed above; the information
required to facilitate change. This is the fundamental aspect of
Metaphon and underpins the rest of the treatment procedure.

Metacommunication is concerned with developing the children's
knowledge that successful communication depends upon the person
who is speaking being understood by those who are listening. We also
show the children that repair, or correction, is the tool which we all
use as speakers to revise and correct our utterances to facilitate understanding. In general terms the metacommunicative and repair aspects
of linguistic awareness reflect the first two of the list of requirements
for reviewing and revising existing phonological systems – knowing
that change is required and that it is possible to make changes. In the
second phase of Metaphon, we develop the children's awareness of the
possibility of communication breakdown and assist them to communicate effectively by encouraging them to make repairs. Their ability to
make such repairs is facilitated by utilising the enhanced knowledge
of the phonological system obtained in the first phase of Metaphon
therapy.

These three aspects of awareness, although given different weight in the two phases of Metaphon, are very closely interrelated in our approach. The nature of this interdependence can be traced in the detailed descriptions of the two therapeutic phases we provide in Chapter 6.

The following examples of the behaviour of normally developing children show that linguistic awareness and other aspects of language develop alongside each other. These observations support our belief that Metaphon therapy, by encouraging specific aspects of this awareness, is an appropriate treatment strategy. The aspects of awareness which are most closely related to Metaphon activities are practising and playing with language and spontaneous use of repairs.

Young children appear to derive an enormous amount of enjoyment from playing with the phonological structure of language. The following was recorded from Anthony, aged 2;6 as he was falling asleep:

Back please / berries [bɛrɪz] / not barries [bærɪz] / barries / barries / not barries / berries / ba ba... (Weir, 1962: p. 108.)

This quotation provides vivid evidence of one young child's ability to pay attention to and manipulate phonological structure. Weir suggests that in this example, Anthony appears to be deliberately practising and perfecting his pronunciation of 'berries'.

Other authors provide examples of language play appearing to have less purposeful intent. The following comes from Matthew, (aged about two) as he was being undressed:

Nolly lolly, nolly, nilly nolly, sillie Billie, nolly, nolly. (Cazden, 1976: p. 606.)

This type of spontaneous rhyming activity has been reported from children as young as 18 months, but it appears to be at its peak between two and three years of age. Children use both real and nonsense words in this type of activity. Sometimes the chaining of rhyming words appears to be triggered by a physical activity, at others it is spontaneously produced. The fact that young children are capable of manipulating phonological structures and appear to derive a large amount of enjoyment and satisfaction from this activity suggests that it is particularly suitable for inclusion in therapeutic intervention, a point we take up again later.

Encouraging children to make corrections and repairs to their own speech to ensure successful communication is an essential aspect of Metaphon therapy. Like playing with language, this ability has also been observed in normally developing children from about 18 months of age. Clark (1978) says that young children will check to see if the listener has understood them and if not they will revise their speech and try again. She cites as an example Brenda, aged 1;5, persisting with and producing seven varied approximations of 'shoe' prior to her mother's recognition of the word.

Clark and Andersen (1979) provide more evidence of self monitoring and repair collected from the spontaneous conversations of 2 and 3 year old children. These authors suggest that repairs to different elements of language predominate at different ages and these appear to coincide with the main stages of acquisition of these elements. Phonological repairs are reported as being the first to occur. These decrease as children get older, and are replaced in turn with a predominance of morphonological, lexical and finally syntactical repairs.

Children will also comment on and correct what other children say, demonstrating their awareness of the correctness or otherwise of certain forms. Iwamura (1980) provides data collected from two 3 year old girls which includes many examples of comment on and correction of phonological, phonetic, syntactic and semantic features of each other's speech. We have also collected examples of phonologically disordered children commenting on their own speech in treatment sessions. For example, Liam (aged 5;3 years) said 'When I say that word (pointing to a picture of a rake) it sounds like lake'.

Although we can provide many examples which show that the behaviour we focus on in the therapeutic situation also occurs spontaneously and naturally during normal language acquisition this does not of course signify that such activities have any role in language acquisition. Furthermore it is important to stress that in Metaphon therapy our aim is to facilitate phonological change by providing the children with opportunities to enhance their phonological knowledge. We offer a theoretically based therapeutic procedure which aims to bring about phonological change through cognitive development as an alternative to techniques which focus on auditory stimulation or specific production targets. We are not implying that linguistic awareness is critical to phonological acquisition, rather that enhancing certain metalinguistic skills may help some children to make phonological changes. However, several authors have put forward theoretical arguments for the role of linguistic awareness in acquisition and we will consider these next.

Metalinguistic Ability and Phonological Acquisition

The strongest argument for a role for linguistic awareness in phonological acquisition comes from those theories which see the process of phonological development as involving children actively discovering how to communicate with others. These theories, such as the cognitive theory of phonological development, proposed by Macken and

Ferguson (1983) and the interactionist discovery theory of Menn (Menn, 1976; Kiparsky and Menn, 1977) appear to presume a role for some degree of metalinguistic awareness during the acquisition process. Proponents of these theories believe that successful phonological development requires children to discover how to communicate with others in their efforts to make themselves understood. Macken and Ferguson believe that phonological acquisition is not automatic and that the child must at some point in development recognise similarities and formulate rules through active experimentation. According to Menyuk, Menn and Silber (1986) this experimentation requires attention to phonemic structure. We take up this point again in Chapter 5 where we consider the social context within which children can be encouraged to formulate such rules.

Certain types of behaviour are cited as evidence that satisfactory phonological development requires active participation by the child. This behaviour includes the selection and exploitation of certain phonemes and avoidance of others by some children. For example, they may demonstrate preferences for favourite sounds, be particularly receptive to new vocabulary which employs newly learnt structures, or they may deliberately avoid using some words (Macken and Ferguson, 1983; Ingram, 1986). In what are apparently attempts to match adult rules, children also demonstrate an ability to combine phonemes to create unique phonological patterns that are not found in their native language. The considerable variation that is known to exist between children in the choice of words they choose to exploit and avoid reinforces the view that they are actively selecting the structures they will work on. This type of activity does appear to depend upon children being sensitive to, and being able to manipulate, the phonemic structure of language in some specific ways. An actively useful role for phonemic awareness in phonological acquisition can therefore be argued.

Clark (1978) argues that an ability to make repairs is essential to enable children to move on from one stage of language acquisition to the next. Clark and Andersen suggest that:

> the awareness of language revealed by spontaneous repairs may play an essential role in the process of acquisition itself. Without the ability to monitor, check, and then repair one's utterances, it is unclear how children go about changing a rudimentary system into a more elaborate one. (Clark and Andersen, 1979: p. 11.)

This suggestion that ability to repair language provides the essential thrust required for language development and that the child is actively involved in acquiring language provides strong support for Metaphon therapy.

There is no firm evidence that phonological play activities have an essential role in the acquisition process. Nevertheless several authors are sympathetic to the possible usefulness of language play in language acquisition. For example, many Soviet psychologists and linguists have regarded linguistic awareness as essential in language acquisition. Chukovsky (1968) in particular believes that children who do not go through rhyme creating activities are abnormal. He sees this activity as providing necessary phonetic practice for all possible sound variations.

If we review what appears to be happening in the phonological play activity, particularly the rhyming activities, several factors appear to support the proposition that this activity may assist in some way in the development of the structural aspects of language. The patterns the children imitate or create observe only phonological rules and appear to serve no grammatical or semantic functions. These productions are not random but appear to involve specific minimal feature changes; the child starts with a known word and manipulates it so that a new word is produced which still retains some of the elements of the previous word. The ability to focus specifically on the form rather than the meaning of language is reinforced by the creation of novel nonsense words to fulfil and continue this minimal feature change. To make these minimal changes to a word or a nonsense word in this manner the child must be aware, at some level, of the phonemic composition of words.

The manner and situation in which these constructions are produced reinforces the view that the child is focusing on practising and perfecting sound patterns rather than communicating. This play usually appears to be a private activity without any apparent communicative function. Garvey (1977) says that the child becomes aware in private of the structural properties of language and takes apart and puts together building blocks of sequences that he or she cannot consciously isolate until later.

To summarise, children who indulge in the type of phonological play activities we have cited above must have some kind of sensitivity to the phonemic structure of language. We cannot yet say whether such activity represents active practice to aid phonological acquisition, or is simply an expression of enjoyment of language. But, it is certain that such activities will reinforce and encourage greater sensitivity to sounds and sound patterns. Therefore regardless of whether or not they are essential for successful phonological development it can be argued that they constitute an appropriate focus of activity in the treatment of phonological disorder. If linguistic awareness does have a critical role in language development it would be reasonable to expect phonologically disordered children to have poorer metalinguistic skills than children whose language is developing normally. In the final section of this chapter we review what is known about the metalinguistic abilities of phonologically disordered children.

The Linguistic Awareness of Phonologically Disordered Children

The surest way of demonstrating an essential role for linguistic aware-ness in phonological acquisition would be to carry out longitudinal studies comparing ability in these two aspects of language from a very early age. Given that relatively few children from the total population present with phonological delay that is sufficiently extreme to warrant parental and professional concern such a study would require intensive study of large numbers of children. The possibility of carrying out such an investigation in the near future appears remote.

There are a small number of observational and experimental studies which provide some information about the ability of phonologically disordered children to make phonological changes in response to lis-tener uncertainty and certain experimental conditions. A few researchers have also compared phonologically disordered and normal-ly developing children's performance on the type of phonemic aware-ness tasks we described earlier. Magnusson (1991) provides a useful review of linguistic awareness in phonologically disordered children.

We will look first at the research which has investigated revision strategies. Studies of the interaction between phonologically disor-dered children and their mothers show that these children are sensitive to whether listeners have understood them, and will spontaneously make changes to their speech output during normal conversation. These changes may include phonetic changes, but there are indications that they do not fully exploit this type of revision. Gardner (1989) com-pared the interaction of three types of children with their mothers: phonologically disordered children, normally developing children of equivalent mental age, and younger children with age appropriate phonological ability. She found that children in all three groups some-times made phonetic and semantic revisions (that is, they altered the structure of a word or used a new word) when the mother indicated to her child that she had not understood. The phonologically disordered group made more revisions than either of the other two groups but showed a preference for semantic revisions. (See also McCartney, 1981.)

Because Gardner's study shows that phonologically disordered chil-dren are able to make phonetic repairs we would argue that in Metaphon therapy we are enhancing and encouraging an ability that they possess but which they do not appear to spontaneously exploit to the full. We have to remember, however, that we cannot isolate the chil-dren's responses from the general communicative situation. The type of responses children make will undoubtedly be influenced by parental input and demands, a point we cover in some detail in the next chapter.

The small amount of research designed to investigate phonetic repair in experimental conditions also demonstrates phonologically disordered children's ability to make such repairs. Such children are found to make significantly fewer pronunciation errors when they are deliberately misunderstood by a listener (Weiner and Ostrowski; 1979). In addition Weiner and Ellis (1980) found that phonologically disordered children who were asked to say lists of words containing potentially homonymous words (for example 'tea' and 'key' which could both be realised as [ti]) were much more likely to make a pronunciation difference between such words when they occurred one after the other. Howell (1989) found that phonologically disordered children made as many attempts as age matched children with superior phonological ability to correct mispronounced words in an experiment which compared the ability of the two groups to judge and correct mispronounced tape recorded words.

These experiments show that phonologically disordered children are capable of increasing the number of phonetic revisions they make to their habitual pronunciation, particularly if they are placed in situations where such changes serve the specific purpose of increasing understanding by the listener. This suggests that structuring the therapeutic situation to encourage such revision, as we do in Metaphon, is a valuable treatment strategy.

Metaphonology, knowledge of the phonemic structure of language, the other aspect of linguistic awareness on which Metaphon focuses, has, as we saw earlier, mainly been examined experimentally by rhyme recognition tasks. Several studies have compared the rhyme recognition abilities of phonologically disordered and other speech disordered children with normally developing children (for example Magnusson, 1983; Stackhouse and Snowling, 1983; Stackhouse, 1985; Naucler and Magnusson, 1984; Magnusson and Naucler, 1987; Howell, 1989).

In our own investigation (Howell, 1989) we compared the rhyming and segmentation abilities of a group of pre-school phonologically disordered children with a control group of normally developing children. Each group contained 21 children, 15 boys and 6 girls. The mean age of the phonologically disordered group (PDG) was 4;2, range 3;8 to 5;5. The normally developing group (NDG) had a mean age of 4;3, range 3;10 to 4;9. The PDG group had a mean standard score of 74, range 53 to 85, on the Edinburgh Articulation Test (EAT) (Anthony et al., 1971), compared to a mean score of 121, range 105 to 149, for the NDG. With one exception, there was no significant difference between the scores on a number of other pre-investigation assessments, including the performance section of the Wechsler Pre-School and Primary Scale of Intelligence (WPPSI) (Wechsler, 1967), auditory discrimination and auditory memory tasks. The exception was the comprehension section of the RDLS (Reynell, 1977), although the mean scores for both groups, PDG 0.3 and NDG 0.8, were above average.

The rhyming task used in this investigation was based on experiments by Bryant and Bradley (Bradley and Bryant, 1978; 1983; Bryant and Bradley, 1985). The experimental items consisted of ten sets of monosyllabic words. Each set contained three rhyming and one rhyming word, for example 'pear', 'bear', 'chair' and 'fan'. The experiment differed from those of Bradley and Bryant in that each word was accompanied by a picture. After introduction and practice items, the children were presented with each set of words in turn and asked to choose the picture of the word which 'doesn't sound the same' or 'doesn't rhyme'. The PDG children were much poorer at selecting the non-rhyming words. The difference between the group scores was significant at the $p < 0.01$ level. There was also a significant correlation between rhyming ability and phonological ability, as measured by the EAT, for the total population.

In the segmentation task, based on work by Zhurova (1973) and Barton, Miller and Macken (1980), the children were asked to say what was the first sound of a series of pictured words. As might be expected, from our discussion of phonemic awareness tasks earlier, this was a much more difficult task for both groups. But once again the PDG children as a group did less well at the task and there was a significant correlation between phonological ability and segmentation ability. Other researchers have found similar differences in performance on phonemic awareness tasks between groups of normally developing and phonologically disordered or other groups of language disordered children. See for example Magnusson (1983), Kamhi, Friemoth-Lee and Nelson (1985) and Bird and Bishop (1992).

So there is good evidence that, in general, language disordered children do less well than normally developing children on these kinds of tasks. However, there is considerable overlap between the metalinguistic abilities of normal and phonologically disordered children. They do not form two distinct groups on the basis of their performance on phonemic awareness tasks, and we found that there were good and poor rhymers and segmenters in both our subject groups. In other words it is possible to have good phonological development and do badly on the rhyming and segmentation tasks, or have poor phonological development and be relatively good at rhyming and segmenting.

On the basis of this evidence we cannot determine a clear directional relationship between phonological proficiency and phonemic awareness. The results indicate that there is some relationship between phonological awareness and phonological proficiency but not the reasons for that relationship; they do not resolve the question of whether phonemic awareness exerts a critical influence on phonological acquisition. There is, however, some suggestion that awareness does influence language development, rather than being a product of development, from an investigation carried out by Kamhi, Friemoth-Lee and Nelson (1985). These authors compared the linguistic awareness of language disordered children with both normal children of the same mental age and with a group of younger normally developing children who had the same level of language ability as the language disordered children. They found that not only the mental aged matched children but also the language age matched children did significantly better than the disordered group on a segmentation task. Research into the relationship between literacy skills and awareness (see Goswami and Bryant (1990) for a detailed discussion) also provides some impetus for continuing to investigate predictive relationships between awareness and phonological proficiency. We need to exercise caution, however, in drawing inferences from research involving the learnt skills of reading and writing and applying them to the developmental process of phonological acquisition.

It is worth looking in a little more detail at individual differences in metalinguistic ability to see if it will help us to further our understanding of the inter-relationship between awareness and phonological disorder. First of all, however, we have to consider the influence of the experimental situation when accounting for individual differences. There are, for instance, a number of reasons why children may do badly on experimental tasks: they may not understand the task or simply be unwilling to co-operate. We saw earlier in the chapter the importance of careful experimental design for successful co-operation from this age group. But even the most attractive task, even though it can increase the chances of co-operation, does not guarantee success. In the last resort we can never be absolutely sure that test scores reflect only ability in the skill we are testing.

One possible explanation for individual differences comes from the probability that children who are described as phonologically disordered constitute a heterogeneous population. It is possible that some of these children may have a specific insensitivity to the phonemic structure of language which will be reflected in their performance in metalinguistic experiments. Such insensitivity may be hindering their phonological development. Other children who do well on metalinguistic tasks, may have the same degree of phonemic sensitivity as children with normal phonological development, but have other constraints, such as motor processing difficulties, which may account for their phonological problems. We look at how Metaphon therapy might accommodate the possibility of diverse explanations for phonological disorder in Chapter 9.

Finally, in relation to the question of individual difference, we have to consider the fact there will always be a multiplicity of individual child variables contributing to task performance in addition to the one which is the particular focus of attention. For example, we saw earlier that chronological age is particularly closely related to success on metalin-

guistic tasks. In our investigation (Howell, 1989), significant relationships were not confined to those between phonological awareness and
ability. We also found significant correlations between age and both the
phonemic awareness tasks. Further indication of the strong developmental dimension of phonemic awareness comes from the results we
obtained when we re-administered the rhyming and segmentation
experiments in this investigation approximately a year after the first
experiment. We found a significant increase in scores for both groups
for both experiments.

Sophisticated statistical analysis is required to determine the relative
influence of different variables on awareness. Most of the investigations
we have cited did not go beyond using group comparison and simple
correlational techniques. In our investigation we did make some
attempt to look at the independence of the relationship between EAT
scores and rhyming and segmentation scores by statistically controlling
for the effect of other variables on the metalinguistic tasks. The association between phonological ability and rhyming ability and between
phonological ability and segmentation ability remained significant in
these statistical tests, demonstrating that in these experiments the association between phonological awareness and ability is relatively strong
compared to the association between awareness and other variables.
We need much more investigation of the relative influence of different
variables on metalinguistic ability in order to advance our knowledge
both of the nature of metalinguistic awareness itself and of the role, if
any, of such awareness in phonological development. An interesting
start has just been made along these lines. Reid (personal communication) has found that chronological age accounts for 70% of the contribution to task performance in a group of language disordered children.

To summarise this section of the chapter: investigation of the phonemic awareness of phonologically disordered children consistently
shows, whatever experimental methods are used, that as a group they
perform less well than normally developing children of the same age.
This suggests that there is some association between metalinguistic
ability and phonological ability, although there are considerable individual differences in metalinguistic ability within this population.

What then are the implications of the results of these experiments
for intervention? We do not know why children with disordered
phonology tend to do less well on phonemic awareness tasks. There is
the possibility that some of them may have a considerable degree of
latent knowledge about speech sounds, but it may not have occurred
to them to use this knowledge to make changes to their speech in the
same way that normally developing children appear to do. Our clinical
experience suggests that this may in fact be the case; several children
who had made only minor or no apparent progress under other treatment regimes made exceedingly rapid progress as soon as we initiated

phonological awareness activities with them. Other children demonstrated in their conversations with us and their parents the degree of interest in sounds that these activities unleashed. Because we cannot explain the relationship between metalinguistic ability and phonological disorder, Metaphon therapy does not aim to target deficits in the child. It was designed and is used as a tool to assist phonological change.

In conclusion, strong evidence exists to support our view that a focus on phonological and communicative awareness is an appropriate and effective intervention strategy for phonological disorder. The activities we use are known to be within the capabilities of this age group. Language acquisition theories provide strong support for a role for some aspects of linguistic awareness in phonological development. Finally, experimental studies show that some phonologically disordered children have poor metalinguistic skills, but that such awareness can be developed if appropriate activities are used. However, using appropriate activities is only one aspect of the remediation process. The ways in which children learn is equally important and we devote the next chapter to examining theoretical issues which help us to ensure that the Metaphon approach enables maximally effective learning.

Chapter 5
Theoretical Basis:
Language and Learning

The Metaphon approach to phonological therapy arose from the authors' wish to ground remediation within a theoretical framework which accounts for both **what** is to be learnt and **how** it is to be learnt. Within Metaphon, as the previous chapter has described, metaphonological knowledge forms the content of the learning as it is our belief that metalinguistic awareness has a major role to play in the remediation of phonological disorder. In this chapter we focus upon the rationale for the optimum learning situation which Metaphon seeks to provide for the phonologically disordered child.

An intervention rationale, such as Metaphon, has to take into account the mechanisms by which children naturally learn their first language, but must also consider the evidence from research concerned with language disorder and acceleration studies. Study of the literature will demonstrate that, at the present time, there is no generally agreed theory of acquisition. Perhaps the most useful position for the therapist is the one that is adopted by Kuczaj:

> ... language development depends on children's processing of input and the influence of past intake (information children have gleaned from past input) on subsequent processing of input. This view emphasises the interaction of information processing and organising predispositions (some innate and others learned) and environmental factors, and at the same time acknowledges the importance of intrinsic motivation in the language learning process. (Kuczaj, 1983: p. 2.)

This view of language learning can be seen to attach great value to children's experiences and even greater importance to their interpretation of these experiences. The vital questions for the therapist are, therefore, what experiences will facilitate language learning (in this case alteration in the phonological system) and how best can the child be encouraged to interpret, or utilise those experiences? It might be expected that the answers to these questions lie, at least in part, in the

76

study of children with language impairment. Can such case studies point the way to necessary, or even sufficient precursors to language development?

Mogford and Bishop (1988) consider the role of variables such as verbal environment, auditory impairment, cerebral damage and neurodevelopmental factors in the context of case studies of language development in exceptional circumstances. They conclude that it is still not possible to be specific about the causes of language impairment. They suggest that the difficulty may lie in the fact that language disordered children do not form a homogeneous group with respect to cause and condition, and that indeed, there may be no single cause of specific language impairment, certain factors acting in combination in the case of a specific child. Thus, for the therapist trying to determine the features of an optimum intervention programme for phonological disorder, studying the literature which focuses on the nature of language impairment is interesting but not sufficient.

More profitable is the research concerned with facilitating aspects of language learning in the normally developing child. This research is concerned with many levels of language, primarily syntax and semantics (referential communication); less often with metalanguage or phonology. Indeed, whilst this book is primarily concerned with the remediation of phonological disorder, it will become evident that the principles which inform the Metaphon philosophy are also relevant to the treatment of other client groups.

The essence of the Metaphon approach is that children should be presented with information they can use within a context which facilitates language development. The remainder of this chapter will consider what these contexts might be, look at the way in which the Metaphon approach incorporates them and discuss how information about the phonological system in general, and the child's own system in particular, can be made accessible to the child.

We will focus upon three contexts: the social context, in which the child learns language actively through interaction with his environment; the verbal context, the influence of the verbal input of others on language development; and the cognitive context, which is concerned with the interaction between cognitive load and language performance.

As will quickly be realised, these contexts are not as distinct as they are presented here but are closely interrelated. Indeed any discussion which separates these factors for the sake of clarity runs the risk of reducing the description of the complex process of language learning to an inappropriately simplistic level. Whilst our argument centres around three contexts, the social context, the verbal context and the cognitive context, these are only three of a wide variety of influences upon language learning, chosen because they represent areas of relevance to remediation in general and Metaphon in particular.

Social Context

Piaget is perhaps the best known proponent of the view that the child has to be an active participant in the learning process (Hartman and Haarvind, 1981). Piaget argued that learning takes place when the child's view of the world is challenged by new information. Other researchers have added a further dimension to this work by studying the effect of the social context on learning (Perret-Clermont and Schubauer-Leoni, 1981; Beveridge and Griffiths, 1983). The social context within which the child explores his or her world is seen as including both the physical environment and the people in the child's world.

Resolving conflicts between early acquisitions and current input is important not only for cognitive development but also for language development. Bowerman (1978) described language development as relying on two interrelated phenomena. Firstly the expansion of the child's linguistic repertoire and secondly reorganisation of the knowledge achieved.

Kuczaj (1983) suggests that language development is best thought of as an ongoing process that involves continual analysis and reanalysis by children as they 'search' for distinctions that have organisational significance for the linguistic system. He relates this view to Rumblehart and Norman's (Kuczaj, 1983) three models of learning: accretion, tuning and restructuring. Accretion refers to the acquisition of new linguistic knowledge, tuning to the categorisation of that knowledge and reconstructing to the relating of these categories to one another. Restructuring has a central role in that it allows for the new interpretation of knowledge, for different and often improved accessibility to knowledge and for changes in the manner in which one acquires new knowledge.

This view of language learning seems particularly attractive when applied to phonological disorder where the essence of the difficulty is the use of sounds in a system which approximates to the adult or target system, and where the knowledge to be explored with the child centres around sound categories. Kuczaj states:

> Experience with the same item in different contexts and different items in similar contexts leads children to create form classes and to later differentiate form classes. (Kuczaj, 1983: p. 2.)

This seems to refer directly to the type of learning problem to be addressed by the speech therapist intervening in a case of phonological disorder.

Support for the notion that children are actively engaged in the acquisition of language, particularly phonology, comes from evidence of rule formation and from the selection and avoidance strategies which children use as discussed in Chapter 4. Within this theoretical framework the child can be seen as progressively revising linguistic knowledge and consequent output to accommodate both processing constraints and information from the environment. Children acquiring language are attempting to solve the problem of how to communicate with other people (Menyuk, Liebergott and Schultz, 1986).

How can the therapist place the child in a context which presents new information, and facilitates tuning and restructuring of both new and previously learned knowledge? As the focus of the learning is language, language is the medium through which exploration must take place. This can occur in several ways: by solitary and/or joint language play; through discussion; or by employing language routines. Within this section the role of play will be considered. The role of discussion will be explored in the section dealing with the verbal context, and the implications of using structured language routines will be covered within the section on cognitive context.

Instinctively therapists have profitably employed the play situation. There seem to be good grounds for this choice of context which will repay further study.

Several authors have pointed to the role of play in developing verbal awareness (for example Cazden, 1983). Kuczaj, in his previously referred to monograph on crib speech and language play, suggests that it is during this naturally occurring activity that children reflect upon newly acquired knowledge and begin to resolve some of the discrepancies that have arisen due to the conflict between this new information and currently ordered knowledge. The consequent tuning and restructuring may take the form both of changing the categories and concepts used to interpret novel information, and of creating new knowledge structures. Language play is a naturally occurring activity which seems not only to be enjoyed by pre-school (Weir, 1962) and school age children (Dowker, 1989) but also to facilitate linguistic and metalinguistic development. If the therapist can capitalise on this inherent interest it seems likely that the child will be maximally receptive to appropriately presented new information.

Kuczaj suggests that at an early age the value of solitary language play lies in the opportunities it provides for children to reflect upon, and experiment with, language in a situation which is free of adult control. This has implications for the clinician who may wish to structure her intervention to allow the child to feel free to play with language. Such play may be a novel experience particularly for the phonologically disordered child for whom sound games may have been less rewarding.

However, the value of language play is not restricted to the early stages of phonological development. In a study of spontaneous and elicited rhyming abilities in 2 to 6 year old children, Dowker (1989) found that the features regarded by Weir (1962) and Kuczaj (1983) as being characteristic of the crib speech of very young children also occurred in considerably older children and in the presence of others. For these children the value of such play could not lie, as had been suggested for the younger children, in sound acquisition, as most of the sounds 'practised' were already in their system. Dowker suggests that there is another function of language play — the development of metalinguistic awareness, a view previously put forward by Pratt and Grieve (1984b). Such evidence strengthens the argument for a component of sound play within a remediation programme which aims to develop metalinguistic awareness.

The following quotation from Schuele and Van Kleek further illustrates the possible influence early sound play development has on the later development of secondary language skills such as literacy:

> Pre-school language disordered children need to be provided with opportunities to engage in language play that will get them accustomed to focusing on the phonological structure of speech and purposefully manipulating sounds of words outside the context of meaningful communication. By developing a foundation of phonological awareness at the pre-school level, the language disordered child may be better prepared for later structured academic tasks that require manipulation of the sound structure of language. (Schuele and Van Kleek, 1987: p. 42.)

How do these findings from the literature, which focus on the child as an active participant in the language learning process, relate to the Metaphon approach? The fundamental argument of Metaphon philosophy is that the child should be placed in a (clinical) situation in which he or she can explore the phonological features of his or her language. Intervention must involve language play which is intrinsically motivating for the child, and provide an exploratory situation where the child can produce and manipulate phonemes without there being a **right** answer. The child and the clinician are equal partners in an exploration of the properties of the sound system.

As the child progresses, the therapeutic situation should offer carefully monitored feedback about the presence of ambiguity so that the child is able to recognise that he or she has not conveyed the intended meaning. Thus the child is provided with information which conflicts with his/her present knowledge, creating a situation in which phonological and metaphonological development can be facilitated.

Verbal Context

Many researchers have studied the effects of communicative interaction on first language learning. As the therapeutic process relies heavily upon verbal interaction this literature repays consideration. Previous studies, such as (Wells, 1978), have indicated that mothers who respond to their children in ways that are closely related to the child's utterance, who use language that is of a similar complexity to that of the child and who accept the child's attempts at words and sentences, facilitate language development. Such work has rarely focused upon development of the phonological system but has been particularly concerned with the acquisition of semantic skills.

One example is the series of studies by Robinson and Robinson (1983a; 1983b; 1985) who looked at the influence of listeners' comments about the reasons for non-understanding upon the child's referential communication skills. They found that children can use explicit feedback about the nature of communication failure to improve the quality of their output. These authors suggest that it is essential for language development that 'conflicts' are created by other people so that the child can appreciate the discrepancy between what was said and what was meant. They argue the importance of communication with others if this metacommunicative awareness is to develop. That is, that the development of understanding about ambiguity (which is a pre-requisite for repair) will be in terms of events in the child's social environment rather than in dawning awareness of uncertainties within children themselves (Robinson and Robinson, 1983b).

These findings have a clear application to the children who are failing to get their message across because they collapse distinctions between sound classes. The therapeutic setting should provide the child with feedback about the reason he or she hasn't been understood. However, this information must be carefully graded to ensure both that it is useful to the child and that the child will not be demotivated (Hartmann and Haarvind, 1981; Clark, 1983). Robinson and Robinson (1983a) themselves found that the optimum occurrence of such feedback was relatively low, suggesting that whilst zero occurrence offers no opportunities for learning, a high frequency might, at best, be of no benefit.

Metaphon attempts to incorporate these findings together with the notion that free, uncorrected play with sounds is beneficial to the child, by providing a multi-level approach to therapy in which the child moves between a free play situation and one in which carefully structured feedback is presented. These phases are not mutually exclusive but are invoked in a way that is directly contingent upon the child's response to therapy. Kuczaj (1983) distinguishes between these two types of language 'practice' in terms of the model that the child is utilising. He argues that when the child produces the model (which is generally the case in the solitary play situation) an opportunity is provided for the child to organise and consolidate the linguistic information recently acquired. It is the function of models produced by others, including the therapist, to be moderately discrepant so that the child can apprehend, and eventually resolve, the discrepancy between the model provided and his or her own knowledge of language.

It is interesting to note Gardner's (1989) findings that the interaction between parents and phonologically disordered children differed significantly from other parent—child interactions within the same peer group. For example, there was a higher proportion of controlling utterances which restricted the content of the child's next conversational turn thus improving the likelihood that the speech disordered child would be understood. This suggests that the models available to phonologically disordered children may be significantly different to those available to other children of their age. Gardner presents evidence that the interaction of the mothers and the phonologically disordered group was comparable to that of mothers and younger children which could suggest that the mothers are providing models they perceive to be developmentally appropriate. Lucariello, Kyratzis and Engel (1986) and Constable (1986) both argue that maternal utterances can structure semantic and syntactic aspects of discourse facilitating the participation of the child by providing surface forms which can be utilised.

Metaphon creates a situation in which appropriate models can be provided by emphasising the importance of turn-taking during both phases of therapy. Thus the focus is not always upon the child's output and the carefully graded model provided by the therapist can aid the reflection process. This is especially so where the therapist engages in discussion which utilises shared knowledge of the sound system: for example saying 'I wonder if my picture will be "bat" or "pat"'. Such discussion which includes words such as 'tell', 'ask', 'hear', 'think', 'wonder', 'sound', or 'word' focus children upon speech and language. Constable and Van Kleek (Constable, 1986) argue that this feedback will aid the development of metalinguistic skills.

This reasoning underlines the importance of reflection in the language learning process. Indeed, as Joan Tough writes:

> The whole business of helping children to use language is more complex than just teaching children words, or helping them construct a story, or immersing them in narrative. There is something about verbal interaction that we have to understand. The child can learn much more than we think from verbal interaction, provided the context is one that has interest for him ... (They need) a challenge to think again. And it is this kind of element which signals "Think again — there's something more" that draws children into the thinking process and makes them reflect on what they are doing and saying. (Tough, 1982: p. 267.)

At the core of the Metaphon philosophy is the belief that the children must have a clear understanding about the nature of the knowledge that forms the focus of therapy and be stimulated to reflect upon their knowledge independently of the therapist. To this end the way that the sounds are to be manipulated is discussed with the children in terms which they can relate to and utilise themselves.

The success of this therapeutic strategy is illustrated by the stories parents tell of the spontaneous comments their children make. These comments indicate that, outside the therapy setting, the children continue to reflect upon and process the information that they have received. These observations, together with the results from phonological assessment (see Chapter 8) reinforce our belief in a therapeutic approach which aims to facilitate the development of phonological skills by increasing communicative awareness.

Cognitive Context

We have previously argued that one optimum context for language learning is a verbal environment in which the mother is responsive to the child's choice of topic and produces speech which matches the complexity of the child's grammatical structures.

However, this is representative of only one style of parenting. Therapists' experience and intuition will allow them to endorse Snow, Dubber and de Blauw's (1982) argument that a parenting style which relies on the routinised use of language can also be productive in terms of language development. The reason for the clinician's recognition of this argument lies in the fact that during the more artificial therapy setting such routines often have to be invoked. It is less easy within the context of a short session to provide an environment which allows contingent responsive talk, particularly if the focus of that talk has to be the one small area of linguistic skill designated as a target for therapy. In such circumstances clinicians have utilised language routines.

These routines are defined (Snow, Dubber and de Blauw, 1982) as situations, or interactions, which are highly predictable, stereotyped or repetitive. Initially the children's responses in these situations are only slot fillers but later these utterances may become subject to a process of linguistic analysis which will result in their acquiring independent meaning in the form of syntactic or semantic representations.

Snow and her colleagues describe the routine situations caregivers and children commonly engage in during the prelinguistic and language learning period. In the prelinguistic period games such as 'round and round the garden', create a set of 'slots' and enable the child to fill them appropriately. These activities can be developed by creating new slots, increasing the infant's participation, distributing the work of playing the games more evenly and by creating a more elaborate game structure. The routine nature of these activities facilitates initiation of communication because the child can independently identify potential slots and use appropriate fillers. Between three and seventeen months the child engages in what Snow, Dubber and de Blauw (1982) term 'instructional games' — 'Where's your nose?', 'Where's mummy?', 'What's that (body part)?' The child is now expected to fill the slots with linguistic responses. Some children extend these games by assuming the role of the questioner. A later routinised language game involves book reading when the mother reads a well known story and leaves slots for the child to fill in.

Why are these routines a productive context for linguistic development? Back in 1962 Weir argued that the well learned form provides the freedom to experiment semantically and phonetically and allows for syntactic embellishments within a known framework. Bruner (1983) developed the notion that infants enter the world of language with a readiness to find systematic ways of dealing with linguistic forms. He argued that the child 'works on varying a small set of elements to create a larger range of possibilities' (p. 29) and quoted Weir's observations of crib speech in support of this belief in the child's 'combinatorial readiness' to find the rules governing communicative behaviours. The implication for prelinguistic and linguistic communication is that it takes place, in the main, in highly constrained settings. 'The child and the caretaker readily combine elements in these situations to extract meanings, assign interpretations, and infer intentions' (p. 29).

More recently, in a similar tradition, Nelson (1986) and her colleagues have explored the nature of the child's cognitive support for the language acquisition process. Nelson argues that the child forms cognitive representations of social interactive events. These representations have been built up to guide interaction in social contexts. The predictability of the routines allows the participants to cope with a greater level of linguistic complexity than would otherwise be possible. Nelson argues that these event representations can be thought of as 'cognitive counterpoints' to routines (Snow, Dubber and de Blauw, 1982).

Constable (1986) suggests that it is easier for children to make use of information if the form of an event is constant. This gives the child the 'cognitive space' to process the more difficult linguistic information — they are able to divert resources normally needed to organise the information towards processing linguistic data.

However, both Snow, Dubber and de Blauw and Constable agree that to be truly productive language learning contexts (routines or events) have to be extended by the mother or clinician. The child has to begin to take a more active role in the routines. This change can be accomplished by the clinician systematically altering the interaction in a way that extends the child's developing linguistic skills.

Constable (1986) applies the theory of event knowledge to the treatment of syntactically and semantically disordered children and argues that:

Language intervention from this perspective involves designing and presenting events that are easily analysable and highly functional for the language
disordered child. (Constable 1986: p. 205.)

How does the Metaphon approach apply these notions to the treatment of phonological disorder? Subsequent to Phase 1, in which the
child has engaged in relatively unstructured sound play, Phase 2 capi-
talises on the value of routines which reduce the cognitive load,
enabling the child to focus upon the phonological contrast he or she is
trying to achieve. It is possible to identify several features of a routine,
or event, which allow the child the cognitive space to use new phonological contrasts. The Metaphon approach includes such features as: a
highly predictable pattern of component actions; a specified subset of
linguistic units (in this case, phonemes); turn-taking routines which
result in each component being repeated several times so that many
examples are provided.

However, this phase of therapy is not independent. It relies upon
the groundwork of metalinguistic knowledge established during Phase
1. The aim of Phase 2 is to provide a context which will facilitate processing of the phonological system. The processing itself relies on the
explicit information about the properties of sounds that the child
acquires during Phase 1, and continues to develop during Phase 2.
Reducing the cognitive load allows the child to stand back from language and see it as a tangible, manipulable object.

Chapter 6
Metaphon Therapy Phases

Phase 1: Developing Phonological Awareness

The challenge for therapists working with phonological disorder is to see beyond traditional clinical learning methodologies to find innovative ways of achieving Grunwell's criteria for principled intervention. She argues, firstly, that phonological therapy should be systematically planned and based on an analysis of the child's speech output. Secondly, that treatment should essentially be concerned with widening the range of sound contrasts available to the child in meaningful communicative contexts. And thirdly, that the emphasis should be on changing sound patterns rather than teaching individual sounds (Grunwell, 1987).

The fact that, for phonological disorder as defined earlier, therapy must focus at the level of the system and not on production, requires new learning strategies. Articulation therapy or production drills will, at best, only be indirectly successful in achieving change as they target neuromotor skills rather than processing. The original challenge for Metaphon was how to influence the child's internal organisation of the phonological system. The earlier chapters have described the solution that we devised and tested, that of enhancing and utilising phonological and communicative awareness. This chapter is concerned with the clinical application of this theoretical approach; how the therapist can develop these aspects of linguistic awareness in a child.

The first step is to clarify what aspects of the child's phonological system should form the focus of therapy. The initial assessment of the child's system, as described in Chapter 3, will provide data that can be analysed to determine which simplifying processes are in operation. The success of subsequent therapy will be determined to a large extent by the accuracy of such an analysis, but certain general principles are common to Metaphon therapy for all children. In the rest of this chapter we discuss these principles and illustrate their practical application.

The Aim of Phase 1

Phase 1 is designed to develop awareness of the properties of sounds and their interrelationships in a motivating setting where the child's successful participation is facilitated. This phase is the most important as it forms the basis for the move to more realistic communicative settings during Phase 2. Phase 1 is the linchpin of the Metaphon approach.

The primary aim of Phase 1 is to capture the child's interest in sounds and the sound system. As discussed in earlier chapters this is a naturally occurring interest in pre-school children with normal phonological development. However, such awareness may have been closed to the phonologically disordered child and it is important to spend time, at this stage of the therapeutic process, allowing the child to realise that it is possible to engage in sound games, an activity that might previously have been found difficult or inaccessible. Optimum results in therapy depend on the child's active co-operation which, in turn, relies upon capturing interest and capitalising on this motivation. In practice, it has been found that many phonologically disordered children are fascinated as they find that they can also 'play' with sounds.

Having engaged the child's interest, the clinician and child explore the nature of the target, or adult, sound system together: that is, the properties of sounds; how sounds differ from each other due, for example, to place and manner distinctions; and the importance, for meaning, of maintaining those distinctions. Later, some awareness of how the child's own system differs from the target system is developed.

Now we will describe the steps involved in Phase 1 of Metaphon therapy and consider how the learning situation can be maximised.

Phase 1 Therapy

Phase 1 therapy is divided into several steps or levels. These levels are slightly different depending on whether the focus of therapy is the remediation of systemic simplifying processes or structural simplifying processes. As there is a considerable amount of overlap, the course of therapy for systemic simplifying processes will be described first with a later section charting the differences relevant for the targeting of structural processes.

The Remediation of Systemic Simplifying Processes

This can be divided into Concept Level, Sound Level, Phoneme Level and Word Level. The child will move through these levels for each of the simplifying processes treated; a positive response to the learning situation at each stage being necessary for transition to the next stage. If the child experiences difficulties at any of these levels there will be implications for the diagnosis of phonological disorder which will be discussed further below.

Concept Level

If sounds are to be discussed and explored with the child, it is essential to ensure that there is a shared understanding of the concepts involved. This is one reason why Phase 1 therapy begins at a level which does not involve sound at all.

The therapist and child play games which involve the vocabulary to be used when talking about different classes of sounds. One of the aims of Metaphon therapy (see below) is to talk to the children about the properties of sounds in a way that they can understand. To allow the clinician and child to make sure that they have a similar understanding of these terms, games such as matching up 'long' and 'short' pairs of socks, or putting bricks at the 'front' or 'back' of a house are used. These activities prepare the child for the use of labels such as 'long' for fricatives and 'whisper' for voiceless sounds later in therapy.

The second benefit of starting at a concept, or non-sound, level is that many of these children have built up a self-image of failing in the speech situation. They are only too aware of the sounds that they cannot say, an awareness which has, unfortunately sometimes been heightened in therapy. Beginning at this non-sound level where they have almost 100% success ensures that the child develops confidence in his or her performance in therapy and therefore has a positive attitude to later therapy which does involve speech sounds.

So Phase 1 therapy begins with the child manipulating toys and games with reference to the properties that are important for discussion of the phonological system. This step in therapy may vary in length depending on the individual child's need, but, even when brief, has been found to be very important.

Sound Level

The next stage is to transfer the notion of these properties, and the vocabulary used to describe them, to sounds. This level allows the therapist to begin by using activities which involve sounds which are not speech sounds. Games can involve musical instruments, noise making toys such as rattles and shakers, and vocalisations made by the therapist and child such as lions 'roaring', cars 'driving' or people 'singing'.

As at Concept Level, the aim is to show the child that sounds can be classified along the dimension which is the focus of therapy. Indeed, any sound can be classified as to whether it is, for example: front or back (an alveolar or a velar phoneme); long or short (a fricative or a stop), or noisy or whisper (voiced or voiceless). In addition to increasing the child's awareness of the dimension itself, the fact that any contribution can be classified (even a grunt can be described as long or short) means that the child's confidence in his or her performance is further enhanced.

Phoneme Level

After successfully responding at the first two levels the child is now ready to move on to activities which involve manipulation of the speech sounds themselves. The child and clinician take turns to produce a range of speech sounds that vary along the dimension in question. Individual phonemes do not form the focus of therapy – all sounds from one class are contrasted with sounds from another, for example a range of stops with a range of fricatives.

The speech sounds may, at different stages, be produced spontaneously or in response to a visual referent (a card bearing a mnemonic of the property in question; for example 'Mr Noisy'). A possible visual referent for noisy/whisper is illustrated by Figure 12. The listener then identifies the sort of sound that is heard ('That's a noisy sound!'). Often, this activity will take place at the same time as a game allowing the listener to have a turn after listening to the sound. The game can often be related to the dimension in question – for example drawing clothes on the 'front' or 'back' of the boy, or feeding the 'noisy' or 'quiet' lion. The game and the sound activity then give many opportunities for discussing, with the child, the feature of the sound class that is the focus of therapy.

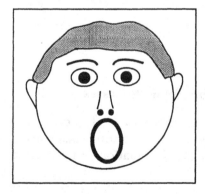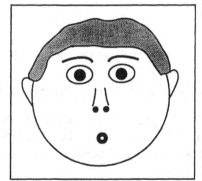

Figure 12 Referent cards, 'Mr Noisy/Mr Whisper'

Word Level

This is the point at which minimal pairs of words differing in the contrast being discussed are introduced. The child is asked to make a judgement about whether the word has, for example, a 'long' sound or a 'short' sound. At this level the child is a listener only but will still be engaged in discussion about the property.

Thus, the clinician may pick up a picture and say 'bee.... I wonder if that's got a noisy sound or a whisper sound?' (see examples of minimal pair pictures for 'pea/bee' in Figure 13). The child may respond with 'noisy' and the therapist may say 'That's right! I wonder if you know any more noisy sounds?' Initially, the therapist may use just one minimal pair to ensure that the child understands the task. Later it may be useful to introduce another minimal pair involving the same contrast (for example bee/pea/toe/dough). The minimal pair picture will have a referent on the back that is familiar to the child from the activities at Concept, Sound or Phoneme Level. This gives the therapist and child additional feedback about the target item.

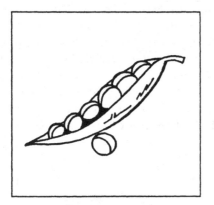 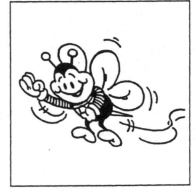

Figure 13 Minimal pair cards, pea and bee

The Remediation of Structural Simplifying Processes

This follows a slightly different course and is divided into the stages Concept Level, Syllable Level and Word Level. However, many features are identical, particularly in the way the information to be learned is presented.

Concept Level

This is almost the same as that described under the remediation of systemic simplifying processes. It serves to introduce the child to the vocabulary which will be used to explore the relevant properties and allow the therapist and child to develop a shared understanding of the concepts involved. However, this level is extended in the treatment of structural simplifying processes to include some of the features of Sound Level discussed above.

For many structural simplifying processes it is not possible to illustrate the concepts involved with activities which involve non-speech sounds. However, this is still possible in, for example, the case of initial and final syllable deletion where it might be useful to contrast, again for example, three notes on the xylophone (representing CVC structures) with two notes (representing either CV or VC structures depending on whether initial or final consonant deletion is the focus of therapy). Thus, for the sake of clarity we have omitted Sound Level for structural simplification processes and have included reference to such activities, when appropriate, under Concept Level.

Concept Level is the only Phase 1 level in the remediation of structural simplification processes where the child is asked to be 'actor' as well as listener for reasons which are discussed below.

Syllable Level

At this stage the child is introduced to syllables which represent the contrast in focus. These may be syllables which form words in English, or nonsense syllables which conform to the rules governing the phonology of English. For example, if therapy involves the remediation of the initial consonant deletion process, V and CV structures are contrasted. The analogy introduced at Concept Level might be animals with/without heads or trains with/without engines. Similarly, if the process to be eliminated is cluster simplification, CCV and CV structures will be contrasted and the vocabulary used for the discussion might involve labels such as 'carts with one/two horses or trains with one/two engines'.

There will inevitably be some merging of Syllable and Word Level. It may not always be appropriate to use nonsense syllables. The decision will depend on the process and the child. In some cases the clinician may choose only to work with syllables which form English words thereby effectively working at Concept and Word Level only. However, in other instances it will not be possible to represent the distinction or contrast simply enough for the initial stages of learning using real words. Then nonsense syllables will be useful.

In the majority of cases at Syllable Level, due to the complex nature of the processing task, the child will always be the listener, only being required to make a judgement about the structures heard. Occasionally, the clinician may work with a child who is able, and happy, to produce nonsense syllables with a particular structure. Obviously the clinician can then capitalise on this. The therapist may use referent cards which can be shown to the child to give visual feedback about the accuracy of the listener judgement. The referent card might have a pictorial representation of the contrast which the child is familiar with – for example, a train with one or two engines to represent one or two consonants word initially (Figure 14) or an animal with/without a tail to represent the presence or absence of a final consonant.

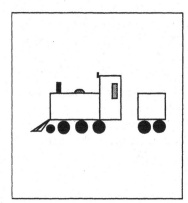 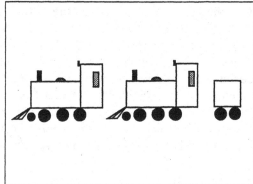

Figure 14 Referent cards, initial cluster reduction

Word Level

This level is the same as for the remediation of systemic simplification processes. At this level again, the child will remain a 'listener'. The therapist will produce minimal pair words and the child will be asked to make a judgement.

Theoretical Basis

It is now appropriate to consider first how these therapeutic activities relate to aspects of metalinguistic activities we discussed in Chapter 4 and second how they incorporate the theoretical learning principles outlined in Chapter 5.

We will look first at why we believe the nature of the information provided in Phase 1 activities, that is specific information about sounds and the features that distinguish sounds and words, is of vital importance in assisting the process of phonological change.

Our belief that children require specific information about the characteristics of speech sounds to make phonological progress is supported by the description of the metalinguistic behaviours of young children. Engaging in the sort of activities we described in Chapter 4 such as playing with rhyme, experimenting with sounds, exploitation of some phonemes and avoidance of others requires something more than simply the ability to distinguish between words. As Kiparsky and Menn (1977), quoted in Macken and Ferguson (1983), suggest:

> At some point the child begins to recognise similarities between classes of sounds and sounds in combination, and to construct rules for relating similar sounds and word shapes and to formulate rules that solve the pronunciation difficulties that are encountered. (Macken and Ferguson, 1983: p. 273.)

In order to gain knowledge about similarities and differences between sounds and sound classes children need to extract information from the speech signal. We will consider the possible process by which they can carry out this activity and describe how we try to emulate this process in the clinical situation.

Our therapeutic approach is analogous with Chiat's (1979) suggestions about the type of information children require for successful phonological acquisition. She observes that the major investigatory focus in phonological acquisition research has centred overwhelmingly on paradigmatic contrasts, that is the features which serve to distinguish one word from another. She says that the child not only has to be able to recognise the differences between words but also has to break up the speech chain to identify individual words. She believes this process of segmenting speech, the syntagmatic aspect of acquisition, is the child's primary task. She says:

> A schematised (and hence oversimplified, though not, I think distorted) view of the child's phonological development is that it starts by ABSTRACTING FORMS FROM the stream of speech and ends up with a store of words WITH WHICH IT TACKLES the stream of speech. It starts with the syntagmatic problem of segmenting a sequence and ends with the paradigmatic problem of distinguishing the elements so segmented. (Chiat, 1979: p. 606.)

So an essential part of being able to distinguish between words is to focus first on breaking up the stream of speech. Chiat suggests that children are aided in this process by paying attention to a variety of acoustic cues, including both supra segmental aspects such as stress and segmental aspects such as vowel length and phonetic features. We suggest that Metaphon therapy provides a clinical correlate for the syntagmatic and paradigmatic aspects of acquisition.

We assist the process in the clinical situation by breaking the task down into small specific progressive stages. At Phoneme Level we do some of the segmenting for the children by using therapy activities that isolate phonemes belonging to specific classes of speech sounds which the child is having difficulty with. These Phoneme Level activities provide the children with essential tools to tackle the next step in therapy, Phase 1 Word Level.

At Word Level the therapeutic task corresponds closely to the paradigmatic task of distinguishing between minimal word pairs which are acoustically very similar. In metalinguistic terms this is a much more difficult task than identifying, classifying and producing phonemes which contain particular features. The child is now required to determine which segment of the words contain the distinguishing features and then to make a decision on which distinguishing feature the therapist has used in the word she produces.

There is, of course, an essential difference between the process of normal phonological acquisition in very young children and the activity of facilitating phonological change in the clinical situation. Our therapeutic activities are designed to provide children with explicit information with the specific purpose of enabling them to consciously reflect about the phonemic structure of language. This process is aided by the use of appropriate verbal labels and visual referents to assist the children to identify and remember the salient features of relevant sound classes.

We can also argue that segmenting the speech signal for the children in the early stages of Metaphon also appears to be a particularly useful strategy when we compare it with the developmental progression of phonemic awareness observed in the experimental situations referred to in Chapter 4. Access to different kinds of acoustic information appears to be required for success in different experimental tasks. Liberman et al. (1974) suggest that segmenting sentences into words presents few problems because words are meaningful units that are required for understanding and using language. These authors suggest that, in turn, syllables are easier to segment than phonemes because each syllable contains a vocalic nucleus represented by a peak of acoustic energy.

More recent work (see, for example, Treiman, 1985), has examined the nature of the syllable in more detail to determine whether there are units that are smaller than the syllable but larger than the phoneme. These units are termed the 'onset' and 'rime'. The 'onset' corresponds to the opening part of the syllable and the 'rime' contains the peak (or vowel nucleus) and the coda (the phonemes that come after it). Words rhyme when they share the same 'rime', so we can see that recognising rhyme corresponds to responding to the acoustic energy peak. Rhyme detection is therefore easier than phoneme segmentation because the phoneme is an imprecise and abstract unit that does not correspond in any direct way with the speech signal. There are no constant specific acoustic criteria to help the child distinguish individual phonemes. They are not produced as separate elements, but are influenced by surrounding phonemes and are transmitted almost simultaneously in a complex continuous signal.

Incidentally, information about segmentation is useful not only because it supports the manner in which we help phonologically disordered children by splitting up the speech signal for them, but also because investigations of the relationships between 'onset' and 'rime' can help us in the selection of target words later in therapy. In particular it suggests that words where the target phonemes occur in word initial position, that is in 'onset' position, are more fully realised and less influenced by surrounding phonemes. This view is supported by Treiman (1985) who found that five year olds are more successful at segmenting initial than final phonemes.

We have used information from acquisition and metalinguistic activities to support our claim that the particular activities we use in the first phase of Metaphon therapy facilitate access to the sort of information that children with normal phonological development appear to access naturally from the speech in their environment. In other words we provide the phonologically disordered children with what appear, to us, to be the most useful tools for bringing about phonological change. We do not make any claims about the possibility that we may, in some way, be tackling the root cause of the problem. This, however, is a possibility worth pursuing further when we consider what is known about the metalinguistic awareness of children with disordered phonology.

Kamhi, Friemoth-Lee and Nelson (1985), the investigators we referred to in Chapter 4, who found that language disordered children did less well on metalinguistic tasks than much younger children with the same level of language ability, also found that the language disordered children had particular difficulty in segmenting words into smaller units. Only two of their fifteen language delayed children, compared to over half of the language aged matched children and 80% of the mental aged matched children, could segment monosyllabic words into smaller units. The language delayed children were also inferior to both groups of normally developing children in their ability to segment bisyllabic words and sentences. If children acquire phonology in the ways suggested by the cognitive theorists it is possible that difficulty in accessing syntagmatic and paradigmatic information from the speech signal will delay acquisition. Support for the view that this difficulty lies at the level of analysis rather than at the surface level of auditory discrimination can be found in Bird and Bishop (1992). We will now go on to consider how the first phase of Metaphon therapy incorporates the theoretical learning principles discussed in Chapter 5.

The underlying learning principles were, for the sake of clarity, grouped as to their implications for the social, verbal and cognitive contexts in which learning takes place. It was stressed that such divisions are extremely artificial in that their tendency might be to hide the overlap that obviously arises. However, such organisation of the discussion allows us to focus on different parameters and assess their relative value and, as here, explore how such features might be incorporated in the therapeutic situation.

Social Context

We have seen that the aim of Phase 1 is to explore, with the child, the properties of the sound system, to show that properties such as frication or voicing are tangible and can be manipulated, and that by such manipulation output can be altered to increase the likelihood that the speaker will be understood. This aim is in line with the belief of workers such as Bowerman (1978), Bruner (1983), Kucsaj (1983) and Rumbelhart and Norman (Kucsaj, 1983), that when learning language the child is involved in a process of discovery – acquiring new information and reorganising his or her system to accommodate that new knowledge.

Phase 1 is designed to provide the child with a motivating environment which gives the child opportunities to acquire knowledge about phonology, about the child's own system and the model system and knowledge about the way in which the phonological system might be manipulated so that utterances more closely match the target.

The activities utilised in Phase 1 have the potential for being motivating on two accounts. First, these games capitalise on sound play which naturally occurs as children develop. As Chapter 4 discusses, children are amused and interested in activities such as rhyming games or 'I-Spy'. Second, the tasks in Phase 1 are couched in the form of a more general play situation allowing the clinician to incorporate games which the child enjoys. One of the strengths of Metaphon therapy is that it is a philosophy, and not a programme. The therapist can use his or her experience of children in general, and of a particular child, to incorporate the aim of learning about sounds in a play environment which is motivating. Chapter 7, which gives examples of activities which have been found to be useful, illustrates the wide variety of situations in which the child can learn about sounds.

An interested child will naturally be a participating child and this is one way in which the next question – How does Metaphon therapy encourage the child to be an active participant? – can be answered. However, Phase 1 is designed to meet this need in several ways in addition to capitalising on naturally occurring play.

The levels into which Phase 1 is organised allow a steady progression of activity which both builds the child's confidence in his or her ability as a communicator and increases understanding of the concepts in question. A good illustration of this is the way in which Metaphon therapy starts by involving the child in games which do not refer to speech sounds. The first two levels of Phase 1 Concept Level and Sound Level are designed to allow the child and the therapist to build up a shared understanding of the concepts which will be used to extend the child's awareness of the properties of sounds. Specifically, the child needs to acquire an understanding of the contrast(s) that must be maintained to eliminate the simplifying process(es) currently used.

The games used at these early levels allow the therapist to determine the most profitable way in which these properties can be shared with the child. For example it might be less useful to use a picture of the front door of a house as a referent for initial consonant deletion than to use a picture of a train with a flag at the front which more graphically captures the linear implications.

When the child has a clear understanding of the relevant concepts the next stage of Metaphon therapy relates these concepts to speech sounds. In the same way that the child has participated at Concept and Sound Level he or she continues at Phoneme Level to be actively involved in the learning situation. Children are then able to participate because they have a clear grasp of the aim of the activities and confidence in their ability to contribute.

Initially, at all levels, the therapist may continually assume the role of the speaker so that the child can participate in the activity without being under pressure. Indeed at some levels of Phase 1, particularly during the remediation of structural simplifying processes, the therapist remains the sole speaker. This is because at these stages the child cannot be expected to generate words containing the appropriate phoneme(s) but is only required to judge whether the word contains the relevant sound. However, the exploration of the sounds and their properties will become joint as the clinician and child begin to take it in turns to be both speaker and listener. This reciprocity has two benefits: first, the child is not always under pressure as the participant who has to produce all the sounds which are 'judged' by the listener; second, the child gains different feedback in the role of listener than as speaker; feedback which reinforces and extends the child's understanding of the way that sounds can be manipulated and combined. Therapeutic activities that involve turn-taking provide one way of ensuring that the child is an active participant in the learning situation.

A further way to encourage the child's involvement in therapy is to present the aim of the learning in terms which the child can both relate to and use, and the next section discusses how the verbal context of the clinical situation can be maximised.

This section has illustrated several ways in which therapy can be organised so that the child is active in the learning process. Chapter 5 provided evidence that such a role for the child not only ensures that maximum learning occurs during the clinic session itself, but also means that learning will continue, and indeed generalise, as the child reflects on his or her knowledge at a later date.

Weir (1962) and Kuczaj (1983) are only two of a number of authors who report instances of children consolidating knowledge gained about language by rehearsing it on later occasions. Evidence from children involved in the first Metaphon efficacy project supported this view of language learning. Parents have provided numerous reports of children spontaneously commenting on the properties of sounds outside the therapeutic situation. Such instances support our belief that, given the knowledge, children will continue to reflect upon sounds and the sound system and our conviction that children who are allowed to be active participants in the therapy process will have the best possible opportunities for gaining such knowledge.

Cognitive Context

The activities involved in Phase 1 of Metaphon therapy are an integral part of the child's exploration of the sound system. Whilst the games are obviously chosen to be motivating for the child the primary consideration is that they reflect the property of system or structure that is the focus of therapy. Thus, there are two constraints on the choice of activities.

First, the games have to be interesting to the individual child, although their complexity must not be such that all the child's processing capacity is diverted to the cognitive task provided by the game. The activity must be well within the child's ability. Second, the game must enhance the learning situation. It can do this by reflecting the properties of the sound contrast that the child is focusing on. For example, if the child is exploring initial consonant deletion the activity may focus on fitting parts to the 'front' of toys – perhaps drawing heads on animals or completing jigsaws. Similarly, if the systemic simplification being targeted is stopping of fricatives, long and short toys can be manipulated to reinforce the property being contrasted. There are many examples of such games in Chapter 7.

If the games are familiar to the child and easily understood, processing capacity can be 'freed up' for the linguistic task which itself will probably require the child to process at the limits of his or her capacity. Thus, keeping the cognitive demands of the accompanying task low will increase the child's chances of meeting the linguistic demands of the situation.

As discussed in Chapter 5, one way to lower the cognitive demands of an activity is to ensure that it is familiar, predictable and routine, leaving the challenge to be provided by the linguistic aspects of the activity. This predictability can also work in the clinician's favour. The chances of the clinician, as listener, being able to detect the child's first attempts at a particular contrast will be enhanced by the predictability of the situation. Within a less structured setting tentative attempts at length or voicing may not be perceived, whereas if, for example, the listener is waiting for one sound which is either voiced or voiceless, any contrast stands a chance of being recognised and can then be accepted and commented on.

As the child's linguistic processing improves it will be possible to extend the demands of the accompanying activity. This can allow the demands on the child's linguistic processing to be further extended to ensure that they are stable before progressing to the next level or phase. For example, the physical demands of the situation could be increased with the child being asked to perform some complex physical activity in order to find the referent which matches the sound heard. Or the memory loading could be increased by involving the child in an activity which includes a delay before the response is given. Such extensions of the basic tasks will be useful for some children but inappropriate for others. Indeed, we have found that for certain children the interest inherent in the linguistic task itself is sufficient to motivate them. They do not require the linguistic processing to be linked to any other activity. The value of the Metaphon approach is that it allows the clinician to structure the learning situation so that it matches the needs of each individual child. What is important is that the child is motivated but not over-stretched, so that all possible processing capacity is available for the necessary linguistic 'problem solving'.

Verbal Context

We have discussed the implications of the social and cognitive context for the learning situation. Now it is time to consider the vital remaining ingredient of the therapeutic setting – the verbal context. How can we manipulate the verbal context to enhance the child's active participation in the learning process?

Chapter 5 considered the role of discussion and comment in learning about language. Therapists have traditionally been aware of the need to structure their dialogue to the needs of the child and Metaphon therapy continues this emphasis. We have attempted to incorporate discussion, graded feedback and opportunities for the child to contribute verbally into Metaphon therapy in order that learning may be maximised.

One of the more obvious ways in which Metaphon has translated these notions into practice is to label the contrasts under focus in ways that the child can understand and use. Such terms differ for individual children depending on the way that different descriptions capture the imagination. For example, voiceless sounds may be attributed to 'Mr

Quiet' by one child but to 'Mr Whisper' by another for whom the quality of aspiration is important. The actual terms do not matter; what is vital is that the labels are meaningful to the individual child and allow each to think and talk about the phonemes and their contrasts.

The initial levels of Phase 1 allow the labels to be negotiated between the therapist and child, and then established so that both share a common understanding of the properties involved. From then on these terms form the basis of the dialogue through which the child and clinician explore the properties of the sound system. Because the child also has access to the vocabulary in which the sounds are described he or she can participate fully in the process of exploration.

In this way, the use of such labels helps Metaphon fulfil its objective of encouraging active participation by the child in two ways. First, these terms allow the child to contribute to, and even initiate, discussion during the therapy session. Second, just as the labels are meaningful to the children, they are also easy for parents to understand and use. Hence, the learning situation can readily be extended to the home situation, and the many examples parents bring of discussion about sounds which they have with their children illustrate this.

A further important point is that this shared vocabulary allows the child to be given explicit feedback about the contrast being targeted. As the work described in Chapter 5 indicated, appropriately presented, children can use detailed feedback to improve the quality of their output. In Phase 1 such feedback will target the nature of the contrast the child failed to maintain. For example the clinician may say 'I'm not sure if I heard a long sound or a short sound', or 'This must be one of Mr Noisy's pictures – Oh! it isn't! It's a picture of Mr Whisper. Tell me again so I can see if I hear a Mr Whisper sound'.

These two examples of responses illustrate the way in which Metaphon moves from a freer to a more structured situation as the child progresses through the levels of Phase 1. Initially the child is encouraged to realise that any sound can be categorised on the continuum of the contrast. However, gradually, as the referents are introduced, the child is placed in the position of being asked to produce a particular class of sound. Similarly, the feedback the child receives will become more focused as therapy goes on.

Whilst allowing the value of explicit feedback, it must be stressed that feedback must always be matched to the child's ability. In the majority of cases all that is required is gentle comment on the features of the contrast: 'I thought I **heard** a back sound' will probably have more positive effect than 'Did **you say** a back sound?'. Also, comment, in contrast to questioning, tends to increase the child's verbal participation. The use of words such as 'think', 'heard', 'wonder' and 'suppose' (Constable, 1986) encourages the child to be an active participant in therapy.

Phase 2 Therapy: Developing Phonological and Communicative Awareness

Phase 2 of Metaphon therapy has three main aims: first, to transfer the metaphonological knowledge gained during Phase 1 of therapy to a more 'communicative' situation; second, to build up communicative awareness (so that the child can recognise when his or her output is at variance with his or her meaning); and third, to develop phonological awareness so that the child can alter or repair output and therefore convey meaning.

These aims are achieved within a therapeutic situation which reflects the characteristics known to enhance language learning. Evidence discussed in Chapter 5 suggests that optimum conditions for linguistic development include situations in which the child is an active participant. These will be motivating for the child and will provide opportunities to reflect upon the sound system. This reflection is aided by discussion which provides feedback about the properties of sounds and the way in which they contrast within the phonological system of the target language.

Whilst the situation must motivate the child it must not be so absorbing as to distract attention from the phonological processing. If the child is processing information at the limit of capacity he or she will need to focus all attention on the linguistic component of the task. Phase 2 requires the child to apply the phonological knowledge gained in Phase 1 to a more realistic communicative setting. The child is involved in complex linguistic processing and, therefore, Phase 2 utilises a language routine designed to lessen the cognitive load so that the child's capacity to process newly acquired linguistic information is increased.

Link with Phase 1

During Phase 1 the child develops metaphonological knowledge; that is a realisation that sounds have properties which can be manipulated, that sounds are contrastive within the system, and that sound contrasts convey meaning. This information is essential for the child in Phase 2 where the focus is on conveying the intended message. The child develops metacommunicative awareness about the extent to which the intended and actual messages match.

The probability of the child being able to convey intended meaning is enhanced by the knowledge gained in Phase 1. Initially, when the child realises that the listener has not understood, the child's increased knowledge of the sound system provides a basis on which to manipulate the utterance. The child is now aware that sounds differ on a variety of dimensions and that changing a feature may increase the chances of being understood. Phase 1 and Phase 2 are not mutually exclusive. Whilst Phase 1 has to precede Phase 2 in order to give the child the necessary knowledge to benefit from the later stages of therapy, the clinician can profitably engage in Phase 1 activities during Phase 2. Such exploratory discussion continues to facilitate the child's developing awareness of the sound system of the language. Indeed, Phase 2 is only meaningful if it is set in the context of Phase 1 work; otherwise Phase 2 activities, and in particular the core activity described below, become devalued because the child's awareness is not primed and therefore the effectiveness of the learning situation is reduced.

Core Activity

The Metaphon approach requires that therapy is firmly grounded in our knowledge of how children learn language, and Chapter 5 discussed the evidence about language learning within three different contexts: the social, verbal and cognitive contexts.

There are many different ways in which clinicians can apply the evidence from the literature to the therapeutic situation. The next section of this chapter will consider how Metaphon therapy incorporates these features using the core activity as an example. First, therefore, it is necessary to specify the nature of this activity. It must be remembered that it is merely a vehicle in which to ground the essence of the Metaphon approach – the therapeutic interaction. The activity itself, essentially recognising and producing distinctions between minimal pair words, could be, and has been, used in many different ways by many different clinicians. However, its familiarity should not detract from the important features of its use in Metaphon therapy or the opportunities it gives for the child and clinician to interact.

The core task we employ is a routine which involves a pile of cards termed 'secret messages'. This label is an easy term of reference for the child, the therapist and the parent, as well as being sufficiently intriguing to establish and maintain the child's interest. The content of the secret messages is determined by the clinician choosing a minimal pair – two words differing in one of the sound properties targeted in Phase 1 (e.g. 'tea/key'). The child recognises, from his previous work at Phase 1, that a change in this property will signal a change in meaning. The therapist places six to eight of these pictures face-down on the table in a random pile. In addition, one of each of the pair is placed face-up to act as 'answer' cards. The 'tea/key' minimal pair is illustrated in Figure 15.

The child and the clinician then take turns to act as speaker and listener. The speaker picks up one picture from the pile and, without the listener seeing, says what it is. The listener then points to, one of the

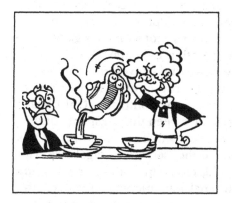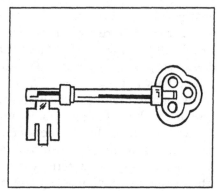

Figure 15 Minimal pair cards, tea and key

'answer' cards, and may also say the word, to indicate which of the two words has been heard. The pictures can then be compared. This allows for both auditory and visual feedback about the match/mismatch between the intended and actual message.

There are obviously several possible sequelae. These will be discussed in some detail because, for the Metaphon philosophy, what is important is not the child's immediate verbal performance but the way in which the therapist uses the situation to enhance the child's learning. At no time does the therapist comment on the child's production of a particular word. All feedback refers to the communicative success of the child's contribution. This is in line with our belief that the nature of the disorder lies not in the production of sounds but in their organisation within the rule system of the target language and therefore that the key to intervention lies in developing metalinguistic awareness.

The first option is that the child, in the role of listener, will pick the correct referent. The therapist can then capitalise on this response by reinforcing knowledge gained in Phase 1, making comments such as 'That's it! How did you know that was the one you had to point to?'. A response from the child which relates to the property in question (for example 'I heard a long sound!') can lead to further discussion. Similarly, in the second scenario, the child who (in the role of speaker) conveys the message appropriately will receive positive feedback which can be expanded into a discussion of other sounds that fall into the same sound class. As mentioned earlier in this section, discussion is far more likely to ensure child participation ('I bet you know lots more long sounds than me!') than direct questioning. The aim is to **explore** the sound system with the child rather than to **teach** the child about sounds.

However, there will be times when the child fails to convey the intended meaning. In this case the listener will select the other minimal pair item. This may stimulate the child to produce a spontaneous repair and as more awareness of the properties of sounds is gained the child will be more successful in manipulating the parameter (i.e. voicing or stopping) which will allow the successful conveyance of the message. This process can be facilitated by the clinician's comments drawing attention to the salient features of the contrast – 'Oh! I heard the one with the long sound. Should it have been the whisper sound?'

At the start of Phase 2 the secret message will be a word only. At this stage it is sometimes useful to combine the 'secret message' task with another activity that interests the child, either preceding or following the core activity of naming the minimal pair picture. However, the extent to which additional activities are employed depends on the individual child. Activities which might precede conveying the secret message include games such as hiding the secret messages around the room, 'fishing' them out of a pond, or finding them in a bag or a sand pit. Activities that might follow secret message production can be as simple as taking off or putting a brick on the appropriate answer card or putting a piece in a form board alongside each answer card. These latter activities have the advantage that the length of the therapy activity can be pre-determined by the therapist regulating the number of bricks etc. to be placed or removed, thus putting a visual limit, which the child can see, on the number of turns. This is particularly useful for the child with a short attention span and/or who may be experiencing some difficulty making changes to their output. In contrast some children may be so fascinated by their newly acquired knowledge of, and ability to manipulate, sounds that they require no other stimulus than the core activity itself. Although the fundamental premise behind Phase 2 Word Level tasks always remains the same, it is the clinician's intuition of the child's learning need which finally determines the way that this therapeutic situation is presented or implemented.

After the child has become successful in conveying the distinction between minimal pair items at the single word level the clinician can extend the activity by placing the target items within sentences as in Phase 2 Sentence Level. The selected sentence is kept constant for both minimal pair items so that the meaning is still conveyed by a single distinction between one pair of phonemes. Examples of such sentences might be:

'Put the picture of seat/sheet in the bucket'.
'Run and jump in the coat/goat island'
(where the islands have the relevant pictures attached).
'Draw a picture of a pea/key on the blackboard'.

It is easy to see how the core activity we have described gives the phonologically disordered child the opportunity to make repairs, in a

carefully controlled therapeutic situation. Such activities are comparable to the spontaneous repair activities that Clark and Andersen (1979)
suggest may be essential to normal phonological acquisition. The activities we use in Phase 2 of Metaphon therapy meet Hewlett's first and
second conditions for phonological change (page 20 this volume):
knowledge that change is required, and knowledge that change can be
made, using the knowledge that the child gained during Phase 1 of
therapy.

We said in Chapter 2 that Hewlett's model allows us to postulate
how phonological change might be taking place in response to therapeutic intervention. We can trace this process by referring to the dia-
gram of the model on page 19. We will provide a brief reminder of the
main points of the model as they relate to phonological disorder.

The Motor Processing component of the model is the key component which puts together the required sequence of articulatory gestures to pronounce a word. There are two alternative routes to this
component, the habitual, automatic, fast route from the Output
Lexicon and a slower more laborious route from the Input Lexicon via
the Motor Programmer.

The slow route to the Motor Processor is used for the child's first
attempts to pronounce new unfamiliar words. The first step is a motor
plan which has to be devised by the Motor Programmer. In order to
devise this plan the Motor Programmer draws information about the
auditory perceptual features of the word from the Input Lexicon which
stores information in this form about words the child recognises. This
plan is in turn passed to the Motor Processor which then assembles the
precise sequence of articulatory features that are required to produce
the word. Once a motor plan devised by the Motor Programmer seems
'reasonably satisfactory' it is used to devise production values in terms
of articulatory features which are then transmitted to and stored in the
Output Lexicon.

The pronunciation errors of phonologically disordered children can
be accounted for because the articulatory feature specification stored in
the Output Lexicon does not always match the auditory perceptual
specification in the Input Lexicon. For example, articulatory features of
place may be neutralised because instead of having a velar place specification, to match the auditory perceptual features of /k; g; ŋ/ in the
Input Lexicon, both velar and alveolar are specified as alveolar /t; d; n/
The result is that 'key' is realised as [ti], 'car' as [tar] and so on.
Hewlett says:

> Once a non-adult representation has become established in the Output
> Lexicon the motivation for later revising it must come from an awareness,
> through intra-personal feedback of the discrepancy, together with some
> kind of experience of discrepancy. (Hewlett, 1990: p.33.)

This quotation sums up what we are attempting to achieve in Metaphon therapy. In terms of the mechanism of the model once a motor plan has been devised pronunciation of a word can only be revised by accessing it again from the Input Lexicon via the slow route. Our therapeutic strategies in Phase 2 are directed towards encouraging the child to devise new motor plans and consequent new articulatory specifications which match the adult target. Change is likely to be gradual and may involve a series of experimental forms before a satisfactory new motor plan is achieved and the new adult like specification transferred to the output lexicon to permanently replace the original specification and serve as the habitual pronunciation accessed by the fast route. Having provided an overview of a possible mechanism of change we can now turn to look at how phonological change is brought about using Metaphon therapy within the context of learning theory.

The core activity for Phase 2 that we have described is not the only example of how the Metaphon philosophy can be put into practice but it is one way in which Metaphon's criteria for the learning situation can be met. These criteria are based on the knowledge we have about how children learn language. Now, let us consider those features discussed in Chapter 5, under the headings of social, verbal and cognitive context, and look in detail, using the core activity as an example, at how Metaphon attempts to incorporate them.

Social Context

The importance of the social context, the environment and the people within it, lies in the quality of the child's interaction with that world. The child is an active learner who must see for him- or herself the result of attempts to communicate. For the phonologically disordered child the focus of learning in Metaphon therapy is metaphonological and metacommunicative knowledge. The child requires a supportive environment in which to develop an awareness of the extent to which his or her system matches the target system – as evidenced by whether or not the meaning has been conveyed.

Metaphon utilises the strategy of conveying the distinction between two minimal pair items. The listener indicates, both verbally and by pointing to a pictorial representation of the item, which 'message' the child has given. The child is then able to match the target picture with the answer pictures and thus gains bi-modal feedback about the success, or otherwise, of an attempt.

Non-judgemental feedback is all that is required to allow the phonologically disordered child to perceive the mismatch between the actuality and his or her intention. This strategy of developing awareness of communicative success in the context of the metaphonological knowledge acquired during Phase 1 meets the requirement of providing feedback which leads the child to progressively revise linguistic knowledge, and therefore output, to accommodate the new information acquired. The core activity stimulates the child's active participation as he or she reflects upon language.

One important feature of an approach which sees the child as an active processor of linguistic information is that change in the child's output will probably not be immediate or clear cut. Children who are constructing their own phonological system will be involved in a learning process in which their performance fluctuates as they assimilate the new information into their systems. The system may appear to have been reorganised, but then may seem to return to the previous state for a while, or there may be evidence of overgeneralisation, assimilation only finally being demonstrated when the system becomes stable again.

The therapist who is aware of the nature of the learning process can accept the various manifestations of the system as a progression towards the target. The learning will be less immediate in its impact than, say, imitation, but will be far longer lasting as it results in a shift in the child's internal processing of the sound system, or motor plan in the terms of Hewlett's model, through increased linguistic awareness.

The belief that the goal of Metaphon therapy is to change the child's internal organisation of the phonological system through the medium of increasing linguistic awareness has a further important implication for the time span of intervention. Therapy based on the mastery of a physical skill, or remediation programmes founded on behaviourist principles of learning, advocate intensive intervention based on the notion that frequent practice will bring about the most change.

In contrast Metaphon's belief that, in the case of phonological disorder, change must be effected through developing linguistic awareness, which has some measure of support from the efficacy study (Chapter 8), calls for a different approach. Children require time between sessions to assimilate the knowledge gained. An example of the reflection that occurs between treatment sessions came from one of our children, Katy, who stopped her father's bedtime reading of 'Baa Baa Black Sheep' to tell him that 'sheep' began with a long sound.

In terms of Kuczaj's (1983) argument, 'timespace' permits post-initial processing of newly acquired information to allow restructuring of the child's knowledge. This restructuring allows further new information to be more easily acquired, allows for the new interpretation of knowledge, and for that knowledge to become more accessible. A time scale which does not allow for this period of consolidation will be wasteful in terms of clinical input.

In contrast to Phase 1, the aims of Phase 2 can less easily be achieved through the free play situation. The child's exploration of the sound system has to be guided so that the requisite feedback about a particular sound contrast can be provided within the time constraints of the therapeutic situation. Thus the second requirement of a Phase 2 activity is that it forms a language routine.

Cognitive Context

Within Phase 2 the child will be processing language at a level which approximates the capacity of his or her phonological system. Thus, it will be advantageous if the child's linguistic performance is facilitated by an activity which embodies the features of a language routine. These were described in Chapter 5 as being situations, or interactions, which are highly predictable, stereotyped or repetitive. These features, which reduce the cognitive load on the child, allow the participants to cope with greater linguistic complexity than would otherwise be possible. The child's participation in these routines can be extended as the linguistic processing becomes easier.

The Metaphon core activity (secret messages) is intended to provide just such a language routine. The task is predictable and repetitive. The children know that the message will be one of two options and that their turn as speaker will always alternate with the clinician's turn. Thus the child's processing of language can focus upon the linguistic, as opposed to the cognitive, demands of the task. It might be argued that the child may find this language routine too routine. For this reason it is suggested that the core activity can be preceded or followed by another activity in the way we suggested earlier. That is the speaker may have to fish for or find a hidden secret message before saying it for the listener. Alternatively, any activity which captures the child's interest without being too distracting can follow the act of passing the message. This activity could be adding parts to a drawing, dressing a doll, building a 'lego' house or placing animals in a farm. Thus, the child's attention and concentration can be kept without distracting from the linguistic focus of the core activity.

The predictability of the language routine can also act in the clinician's favour. If the child's utterance is liable to be one out of two options, the listener will be attuned so that it will be possible to catch small alterations in the child's output which indicate a move towards the adult realisation of a phoneme. Such small adjustments might well be missed in a less structured situation.

As the child's ability to make a linguistic contrast improves and stabilises the language routine can be extended. One way in which the core activity has been extended is to place a minimal pair which embodies the contrast within the context of a sentence. This means that the child has to maintain the distinction within continuous speech but continues to restrict the nature of the processing task by ensuring that the meaning is still carried by the minimal pair contrast and not by other differences between utterances. In addition, the complexity of the task can be varied in terms of the position of the minimal pair within the sentence. The level of difficulty posed by different contexts will depend on the individual child's system.

A further way in which the core activity can be extended is to present the child with the need to make a three- or even a four-way distinction. These stimuli may all be contrastive (for example comb/coat/coke) or may form two minimal pairs (contrasting sea/tea and shoe/two within the same session). Again, the choice within the options will depend on the individual child's phonological system and response to therapy.

The final aim will be to move in controlled stages towards a situation in which the child and therapist can discuss sounds and the reason for communication breakdown. The increased metalinguistic awareness the child gains during therapy makes this approach feasible. It is easy to see how a comment such as 'I know you say "wego" but I say "wego"' can lead to discussion of the reasons for the loss of contrast. However, such discussion is only possible and meaningful with a child who has developed sufficient reflective ability.

It cannot be stressed too often that the examples quoted here are only a selection of ways in which the inventive clinician can manipulate the therapeutic situation. The important feature is that a child's linguistic performance is maximised by the reduction of the cognitive demands of the activity.

Verbal Context

The Clinician's Role

The verbal input from the therapist or the caregiver is a vital part of Phase 2. The way that the core activity is presented, and the manner in which the child's utterances are accepted and responded to, are essential to the efficacy of the core activity. It is the prominence of Phase 1 and the resulting nature of the interaction in Phase 2 which gives Metaphon its specific emphasis.

Feedback is given at all stages in Phase 2 therapy. Initially, the child is given feedback as to whether or not the message has been conveyed. At this stage the feedback never focuses upon the child's production of the target phoneme, but is concerned solely with communicative effectiveness. The aim is to signal to the child when there is a discrepancy between the intended and actual message conveyed.

However, the strength of the Metaphon approach lies in the fact that the child who fails to maintain the distinction which conveys the meaning will, in addition to receiving feedback about communicative effectiveness, have some knowledge of how to repair the communicative breakdown. This awareness will have originated in Phase 1 and will be reinforced through discussion during Phase 2.

The discussion within Phase 2 may have several purposes. Examples from several different children/sessions follow:

1. To give feedback about communicative effectiveness:
   (Picking up a picture of a fan)
   'Your message is "fan" – am I right?'
   (Picking up a picture of a bat)
   'The noisy one "bat"? – Oh! it's the quiet one "pat", I see.'

2. To reinforce information gained during Phase 1:
   'It was "tar" the front one! Do you know any other front sounds?'
   'I bet you know more long sounds than me. I can think of /s/ – are there any more?'
   'How did you know it was "key"? Did you hear the back sound ..../k/?'

3. To discuss failure explicitly:
   'That's funny! I thought you said "tick". It was "stick", was it? The two horse one. I will listen hard next time and see if I can hear two sounds.' (Where words with clusters in syllable initial position are referred to as carts with two horses as opposed to words which begin with an individual phoneme – carts with one horse.)
   (child: /sss-to/) 'Do you know, I heard "sew" and "toe" that time! ...... Which one was it?'

Referring to sounds in a way which allows children to discuss them allows specific exploration of the reasons why a child has failed to convey meaning. As discussed in Chapter 5 there is evidence that graded feedback about the reasons for communication breakdown is an important feature in the language development process. However, this should obviously take place within the context of a supportive situation as a low incidence (as opposed to a high, or no incidence) appears to be the optimum level of feedback that children can use.

The Metaphon core activity is one example of a supportive environment created firstly, by the nature of the clinician's verbal responses, and secondly, by the turn-taking and minimal pair features. The latter means that, due to the turn-taking convention, the child will only be required to give a verbal response in 50% of the turns, and as there will be success with at least one of the minimal pair items (the one to which the child collapses the distinction) the child will only be attempting the more complex processing task in 25% of the total turns. This fact, coupled with the non-judgemental feedback advocated, ensures that the communication situation remains highly motivating for the child.

In these ways the verbal context can combine with the learning environment to develop the linguistic awareness so necessary for linguistic

development. Clinician/child interaction within Phase 2 should be characterised by the use of those terms which encourage reflection.

The Child's Role

The core activity has been used as an example of the way in which therapy can translate learning principles into practice. The advantage of a
philosophy, such as Metaphon, as opposed to a more directive remediation **programme**, is that the responsibility for applying the theoretical notions lies with the clinicians. They alone can incorporate the
theory into a learning situation appropriate for an individual child.

A further illustration of this vital emphasis arises when the possible
responses to the therapeutic situation are considered. Within an
approach such as Metaphon there is no pressure to complete the task
'correctly' or even to complete it at all. The therapy sessions (and within them the specific activities) exist solely to provide an opportunity to
explore the sound system with the child. Any response produced by
the child, and almost any situation arising, can be used in the further-
ance of Phase 2's aims of developing metacommunicative and
metaphonological awareness to facilitate reorganisation of the phonological system.

To examine this further we will consider a selection of examples
(provided by courtesy of Anne Hill) of occasions when children did not
respond in the anticipated way to Metaphon therapy. The examples
illustrate how the clinician can use these responses to further the aims
of therapy. Careful analysis of these responses provides a window onto
the child's phonological system which allows remediation to be targeted specifically towards the mismatch between the target system and the
child's system.

Example 1

This example concerns a child (Tim, 4;7) who made a contrast between
the minimal pair items which did not resemble the adult or target contrast – a relatively common occurrence. Tim had progressed in Phase 2
from collapsing the distinction between 'sea' and 'ee' (represented pictorially by a mouse) to [i] and had begun to use [hi] for 'sea'. /h/ represents a phoneme in the same class as /s/ (fricative). This was accepted
by the clinician as a contrastive alternative phoneme because Tim had
managed to create a contrast between a V and a CV sequence even
though the C was not the target fricative.

This case illustrates how the child initially needs positive feedback
to indicate that he or she has achieved a distinction between the minimal pair items. The feedback can then be changed to encourage the
child to reflect further on the exact nature of the required contrast.

Having made a distinction between 'sea' and 'ee' Tim was then encouraged to think further about the contrast by comments such as 'Yes, that one's got the engine sound on the front hasn't it? That's right, "sea" there's that engine sound', (where the term 'engine sounds' had been used to verbalise the difference between CV structures – trains with engines – and V structures – trains without engines).

The clinician noted that it was possible to see Tim experimenting with the articulatory posture required for /s/ even though she had at no stage drawn attention to this. Several secret messages later he produced /s/ following the therapist's response which included the word 'sea'. The clinician then attempted to extend his contrast system using the following strategy:

> When Tim said [hi] she moved her hand away from the picture of 'ee' towards 'sea' but feigned confusion about whether the message was actually 'sea'. Tim then produced [s-hi] and on a subsequent turn a closer [s-i].

This was the first occasion on which Tim had used a fricative in word initial position and it appeared to be contingent upon his growing awareness both that an 'engine sound' was required and of the implications of listener confusion. If the clinician had failed to accept [hi] in the first place, or accepted it without encouraging Tim to reflect further, it seems less likely that he would have attempted /si/ as the target contrast.

This illustrates how the clinician's responses can guide the child's exploration of the sound system. In the week following the session reported above, Tim told his mother with apparent pleasure, that 'spot' was like 'pot' with an 'engine sound' – evidence of the learning that had taken place.

Example 2

We have previously discussed the 'variable experimentation forms' (Macken and Ferguson, 1983) which children produce as they search for a solution to their output difficulties. These forms may include sounds which do not occur in the native language. Leonard comments that:

> models of phonology which view the child as an active participant in the acquisition process seem to be alone in allowing for the possibility ... that children may arrive at phonological solutions with sounds or suprasegmental features not in the language they hear. (Leonard, 1985: p. 9.)

This example discusses one way in which this behaviour might be dealt with within the framework of Metaphon therapy.

Chris (5;5) worked on two processes one after the other in therapy – stopping of affricates and gliding of /r/ → [l]. During Phase 2 therapy for each of these processes Chris devised his own contrastive phoneme to deal with the requirements of the task. In the elimination of the sim- plifying process stopping of affricates, the property focused upon is length. The child learns to manipulate this parameter in order to con- vey meaning. In Phase 1 Chris had indicated awareness of this property and had shared with the clinician knowledge of phonemes that demon- strated the long or short concept.

However, during Phase 2, Chris initially found it difficult to repair in the situation of listener confusion. If the listener selected the 'wrong' minimal pair item, Chris could not manipulate the element of length to convey his meaning. The clinician dealt with this by encouraging him with comments such as 'That was "tin" – the one with the short sound. Do you think we might need the one with the long sound – "chin"?' Chris then began to use a phoneme which was difficult to transcribe to convey length when producing contrast 'chin' (v. tin), or 'chop' (v. top). However, there was a definite attempt at creating length. Whilst he was producing [ti] for 'tea' he was using a phoneme which could perhaps be described as /t/ + frication + /in/ to represent the affricate. This was accepted as a contrast and as Chris continued to be involved in the guided discussion and reflection of Phase 2 his output gradually approximated the target phoneme.

Chris demonstrated similar experimentation with the phoneme /r/. This had initially been verbalised as a 'Mr Grumble' sound and he had 'growled' his way through Phase 1. During Phase 2 the growling per- sisted rather longer than the clinician had expected. It was accepted as a contrast to /l/ and at first Chris maintained the distinction by produc- ing 'lake' and [rrrrr] 'lake'. As Phase 2 progressed and more feedback was given about the target phoneme Chris's output approximated this more and more closely.

The therapist has to be aware that there might possibly be this pro- gression through variable forms within the learning process, thus allowing verbal interaction with the child to be altered accordingly. This progression should also be explained to relevant caregivers who might otherwise fail to recognise the emerging shift in the child's sys- tem. The clinician's specialist knowledge is vital for helping others to understand the complex subtleties of the remediation process.

Example 3

Tim, from example 1, also provides an instance of the way the clinician might deal with the small but practical problem recognised by John (5;8) who said (in exasperation) 'I could just **show** you the right one'. Children who are aware that they might not always be understood will also be aware of supplementary ways in which they can convey meaning. These children may point to the answer card whilst conveying the secret message (as Sarah said, pointing: 'That one there, silly!') or may gesture the message.

When Tim was initially trying to convey the difference between /i/ (the mouse sound) and 'sea' and the clinician didn't understand he said 'No, [i]' then gestured swimming and said 'You know [i]'. When this behaviour first occurs it is obviously important for the therapist to acknowledge that meaning has been conveyed. The alteration to the learning situation can then be circumvented by introducing the additional element of the listener either closing their eyes when the message is being conveyed, or even turning around. These features can be incorporated naturally as they can add to the element of 'secrecy'. This illustrates the way in which Metaphon therapy calls for clinicians to be flexible and creative in adapting the therapeutic situation to suit the learning needs of the child.

Example 4

Having become active participants in Phase 1 and been able to convey the distinction between the minimal pair items at Phase 2 Word Level, some children find transitory difficulty in moving on to Sentence Level. This is a further instance of the way in which the clinician's verbal interaction can clarify the demands of the task for the child so that participation is possible. When the child says 'key' instead of 'Put the key in the bag', comments such as 'You've told me the message – now what shall I do with it?' generally stimulate the required response.

Example 5

Therapy can also serve a diagnostic function. The child's response to a particular phase can confirm or question a diagnosis. This is particularly important in the case of children who present as complex cases, perhaps with very restricted output or co-operation. If a child fails to attempt to make a contrast between the minimal pair items during Phase 2, despite obvious listener confusion, the clinician must examine possible reasons and adjust the progress of therapy accordingly.

One possible explanation is that the child has not gained sufficient awareness of the properties of sounds, the parameters along which they differ, and the way in which sounds can be manipulated, during Phase 1. In this case the therapist should return to Phase 1 type activities and note the child's response. The observation that the child's participation in Phase 2 type activities can be enhanced in this way provides additional support for our contention that Phase 1 is the vital phase in therapy. However, if the child experiences persistent difficulty, with or without increased awareness of sounds, the clinician will need to question the diagnosis of phonological disorder and should begin to suspect that the disordered phonology arises from some other physical, sensory, neurological or cognitive cause.

The child's response to remediation should give some clue as to the nature of the underlying disorder which can be confirmed by further assessment. For example, it might be suspected that the child who fails in the role of listener has a sensory problem which prevents reception or interpretation of the speech signal. In contrast, the child who is obviously aware of listener confusion but cannot produce a meaningful alteration in the target phoneme, may have an articulatory deficit which precludes success in this learning situation.

Whilst the child's performance might lead the original diagnosis of phonological disorder to be questioned during Phase 1, some difficulties do not become apparent until the child is required to function within the communicative setting; specifically when they are asked to combine phonemes into words. The clinician must always be alert to interpret clues from the child's response to therapy, searching for reasons for lack of success within the way the learning situation is organised to take account of the child's underlying strengths and constraints.

Chapter 7
Metaphon Therapy: Practice

The previous chapters have discussed the theoretical principles on which Metaphon is based and have shown how the therapeutic philosophy was devised to incorporate these principles. This section deals with more practical issues involved in the organisation of a course of Metaphon therapy.

Organisation

Firstly, let us consider how the levels of Metaphon therapy might be translated into temporal terms. As therapy for systemic and structural processes is slightly different we will separate the two and look first at a hypothetical plan for the week-by-week organisation of Metaphon therapy aimed at the elimination of a systemic simplification process (Table 2). This plan is a hypothetical one formed after analysis of the data from the efficacy study reported in Chapter 8 (as is the plan described for the remediation of structural simplifying processes below).

We stress that these plans are hypothetical and merely form a base from which decisions can be made about the course of an individual child's therapy. Many factors need to be taken into account in the real life situation not least the child's motivation, attention span, learning ability and, of course, success rate. However, these composite plans, based on experience gained during the supporting research, provide a basis from which to work. Such guidelines, interpreted in the light of the individual child's abilities, give the therapist an indication of the time treatment may take. This information can be useful for therapists new to the Metaphon approach and for parents.

The hypothetical plan for the remediation of structural simplifying processes, (Table 3) differs from that for systemic simplifying processes in two ways: the levels themselves are different and the time allotted to each of the stages is changed. This alteration is due to the fact that it is not generally realistic to ask children to be 'speakers' during the Phase

Table 2 Therapeutic plan for systemic simplification processes

Phase 1
    Session 1
        Concept/Sound Level
        Concept/Sound Level
        Phoneme Level*
    Session 2
        Concept/Sound Level
        Phoneme Level*
        Phoneme Level
    Session 3
        Phoneme Level
        Word Level*
        Word Level*
    Session 4
        Phoneme Level
        Word Level*
        Word Level*
Phase 1 and 2
    Session 5
        Word Level* (Phase 1)
        Word Level (Phase 2)
        Word Level (Phase 2)
    Session 6
        Word Level* (Phase 1)
        Word Level (Phase 2)
        Word Level (Phase 2)
Phase 2
    Session 7
        Word Level
        Sentence Level
        Sentence Level
    Session 8
        Sentence Level
        Sentence Level
        Sentence Level

* Therapist only speaker

1 activities which develop the necessary linguistic awareness of structure; for example, at Syllable Level, to produce nonsense syllables with
the required structure. Thus, in keeping with Metaphon's aim that the
child be active in the learning process, Phase 1 itself is curtailed with
the extra sessions being transferred to sessions which combine Phase 1
and Phase 2 activities.

To illustrate the relatively arbitrary nature of these plans we will cite
the examples of children who were subjects in the efficacy study
reported in Chapter 8 and whose responses to therapy caused the out-

Table 3 Therapeutic plan for structural simplification processes

Phase 1
   Session 1
      Concept Level
      Concept Level
      Syllable Level*
   Session 2
      Concept Level
      Syllable Level*
      Word Level*
Phase 1 and 2
   Session 3
      Syllable/Word Level* (Phase 1)
      Word Level* (Phase 1)
      Word Level* (Phase 2)
   Session 4
      Syllable/Word Level* (Phase 1)
      Word Level* (Phase 1)
      Word Level* (Phase 2)
   Session 5
      Word Level* (Phase 1)
      Word Level (Phase 2)
      Word Level (Phase 2)
   Session 6
      Word Level* (Phase 1)
      Word Level (Phase 2)
      Word Level (Phase 2)
Phase 2
   Session 7
      Word Level
      Sentence Level
      Sentence Level
   Session 8
      Sentence Level
      Sentence Level
      Sentence Level

*Therapist only speaker

line to be adapted in different ways. In many of the cases quoted the time was reallocated to, or from, other stages of the therapeutic process.

Ted (4;2)

The second process to be targeted in therapy for Ted was the structural simplification process initial consonant deletion which primarily affected fricatives. (See below for discussion of remediation of first process.)

For the second process, Ted's sessions were organised as follows:

Phase 1	Phase 1 and 2	Phase 2
6 (100%)	1	5 (0%)*
(2)	(4)	(2)†

*The figures in brackets represent the monitoring trial scores at the end of each stage of therapy, the aim being 0% occurrence of a process; † these figures represent the guideline number of sessions presented above.

During the first two sessions, Ted was obviously uninterested. The clinician had difficulty determining the reason for this, querying, amongst other explanations, tiredness and/or failure to target the explanation at the right level for Ted. At the beginning of the third session Ted's mother reported that he had not wanted to attend and had said that he 'didn't understand'. During this session he appeared more motivated although his responses still seemed to indicate that he did not have a grasp of the ideas presented. The clinician then decided that Ted perhaps required a more concrete illustration of the concepts involved and decided to go straight to Phase 1 Word Level where pictures could be used to illustrate minimal pair items. During this fourth session Ted was motivated and his performance improved. By the fifth session he was 95% correct when he judged the presence or absence of the initial consonant in the clinician's single word output.

This case illustrates the importance of presenting the learning in a way that the child can use. Ted's satisfactory completion of this course of therapy was dependent upon the clinician finding an understandable way to explain the contrast to Ted. In this case visual cues were useful. Another child, as discussed in Chapter 6, might need different terminology; for example, the altering of 'Mr Quiet' to 'Mr Whisper'.

Whilst not strictly relevant to this heading it is worth considering here the further course of Ted's exploration of this process. As can be seen from the chart at the beginning of this case study the allocation of time to the stages Phase 1 and 2 and Phase 2 was slightly different from what might have been expected. This division was prompted by Ted's response to therapy. As we have outlined, he eventually gained an awareness of sounds during the stage which involves Phase 1 activities alone. Indeed his awareness and interest in sounds was, by the seventh session, far in advance of his ability to produce the contrast. He would begin each session by telling the clinician of the words he had found that week which began with an 'engine sound'.

In taking account of this ability the clinician decided to concentrate on Phase 2 activities which gave him the opportunity to be speaker and put him in situations which would stimulate revision and repair. The score on the monitoring assessment administered during the final session revealed that the percentage occurrence had dropped to 0%.

Sam (4;4)

Sam also spent rather longer at Phase 1 than was expected but for quite different reasons to Ted. His therapy programme for the first process treated, velar fronting, involved more sessions at Phase 1 but no additional sessions at the two other stages:

Phase 1	Phase 1 and 2	Phase 2
6 (100%)	2	(0%)*
(4)	(2)	(2)†

*Figures in brackets represent the monitoring trial scores at the end of each stage of therapy; aim 0% occurrence of a process; † these figures represent the guideline number of sessions presented above.

From the first session Sam enjoyed therapy and seemed fully aware of the contrast which was being explored. He appeared to know that there were occasions when he needed to maintain this contrast and there was evidence of active reflection on the concepts presented. Despite this, Sam obviously found it very difficult to produce any back sounds when it was his turn to be speaker. By the fifth session he was only able to produce one after several practice attempts. Sometimes, despite all his efforts he did not succeed and his awareness of this was clear. When prompted by the clinician saying: 'Oh, I think that's a front sound. I know a back sound /k/'. He replied 'That's what I was saying'. However, when the clinician entered the waiting room at the beginning of the sixth session, Sam was spontaneously producing [k..k..k] as he played and when the therapist remarked on this, he told her that it was a 'back sound'. His mother reported that he was engaging in a lot of similar language play at home.

From then on Sam was able to participate fully in remediation and after the eighth session the occurrence of velar fronting had moved from 100% (initial monitoring trial) to 0% (final monitoring trial).

Jack (3;8)

The first process to be remediated was syllable initial voicing. Jack's progression through therapy differed from the hypothetical organisation presented as he spent longer at the stage which involves a combination of Phase 1 and Phase 2 activities after which his reassessment showed that occurrence of the process had dropped to 0% and so therapy was discontinued without completing the stage involving just Phase 2 (Sentence Level).

Phase 1	Phase 1 and 2	Phase 2
4 (100%)	4 (0%)	0*
(4)	(2)	(2)†

*Figures in brackets represent the monitoring trial scores at the end of each stage of therapy; aim 0% occurrence of a process; † these figures represent the guideline number of sessions presented above.

During the Phase 1 stage Jack was generally accurate in the role of listener. When he was a speaker he produced stops but no fricatives. However, throughout the sessions which provided Phase 1 therapy alone it was difficult to tell if he really understood the concepts involved or whether there was a large element of guesswork. The therapist referred to his behaviour as 'impulsive'. This type of response initially continued as therapy moved into the stage which includes Phase 1 and Phase 2 activities but after two sessions at this stage, a change was noted. During Phase 2 activities Jack began to show evidence of spontaneous reflection and monitoring. Before the listener gave any feedback he would alter his output so that it more closely approximated the target form. For example, in a game where he was required to ask the listener to 'Stick the coat/goat on the board' he said 'Go and stick the goat – no, not that one – the coat' **before** the listener responded.

On reassessment the monitoring trials showed that the occurrence of this process had dropped to 0% and thus therapy was discontinued. Jack's newly found ability to reflect and to initiate repair strategies had led to generalised improvement rendering more work at Phase 2 Sentence Level unnecessary. (More details of Jack's progression through therapy are given later in the chapter.)

Ted (4;2)

The first process remediated was velar fronting. Ted's response to therapy was good from the start. By the end of the third week his mother was reporting that Ted was initiating activities at home in which he said words and she had to comment on the front/back dimension. He also asked his mother to guess which item of a minimal pair of words he said.

After three weeks Ted moved on to the stage where Phase 1 and Phase 2 activities are presented. In therapy there were many instances of spontaneous repair in response to listener feedback and the therapist and mother discussed how to facilitate the use of repair strategies when Ted had trouble making himself understood at home. During the third and fourth sessions at the Phase 1 and 2 stage Ted began to appear bored and his mother commented that 'he feels he knows it all'. Reassessment showed that the process occurrence had dropped to 20%

and therapy for the first process was therefore discontinued.

Ted's progression through the therapy stages was as follows:

Phase 1	Phase 1 and 2	Phase 2
3 (100%)	4 (0%)	0*
(4)	(2)	(2)†

*Figures in brackets represent the monitoring trial scores at the end of each stage of therapy; aim 0% occurrence of a process; † these figures represent the guideline number of sessions presented above.

This reflects his ability to respond to therapy aimed at encouraging metalinguistic awareness, but also illustrates the importance of motivation for a successful outcome.

Mark (3;10)

Mark's therapy plan was very similar for both processes targeted:

First Targeted Process: Stopping of Fricatives

Phase 1	Phase 1 and 2	Phase 2
4 (100%)	4	1 (0%)*
(4)	(2)	(2)†

Second Targeted Process: Liquid/Glide Simplification

Phase 1	Phase 1 and 2	Phase 2
4 (80%)	4	1 (0%)†
(4)	(2)	(2)†

*Figures in brackets represent the monitoring trial scores at the end of each stage of therapy, aim 0% occurrence of a process; † these figures represent the guideline number of sessions presented above.

During remediation of the first targeted process Mark was very quick to understand the concepts involved. Indeed, at the beginning of the second session, when the clinician asked him what sort of sounds they were 'doing' during the last session, he immediately said '/s/ – a long sound'. When Phase 1 Word Level was introduced there were many instances of spontaneous repair.

During the stage when Phase 1 and Phase 2 activities were carried out Mark's mother reported instances of repair at home. He had said [boʌ] for 'four' and she responded that she thought it was meant to be a long sound at the start and not a short sound /b/ and Mark produced [foʌ]. In therapy, Mark reacted to listener confusion by repairing the utterance. When Mark was reassessed at the end of the first session in the

Phase 2 stage, occurrence of stopping of fricatives had dropped to 40% and therapy was discontinued.

A similar pattern was seen for the second targeted process. By the end of the stage when Phase 1 activities alone were used Mark was heard and reported to engage in solitary sound play, practising the elements of the contrast (i.e., repeating 'white', 'white', 'light', 'white' to himself). His case notes report that /l/ was described as the 'friendly sound' ('Mr Friendly' is happy and he sings la, la, la) and provide an interesting example of the hierarchical cueing used to move Mark towards spontaneous repair. The cueing sequence for a word in which gliding occurred was as follows:

Initially, 'Do we need a friendly sound for that word?'
Then, 'The what?' (where 'what' referred to the item starting with /l/)
Then 'the ...?'

Then the clinician merely looked at Mark when the item was produced. Eventually, Mark repaired spontaneously. This cueing hierarchy was successful during one session. When Mark was reassessed during the first session at the Phase 2 stage, the occurrence of the process had dropped to 0% and therapy was discontinued.

This case illustrates the importance of systematically moving through the different phases of remediation with a child even if he or she appears to grasp all relevant concepts immediately. Awareness of phonological aspects has to be matched with communicative awareness which helps the child see when repair is necessary.

Summary

These cases have been described to underline the point that, whilst it is possible and helpful to provide a hypothetical plan for remediation, each child will require to have that plan adapted if the learning opportunities provided by therapy are to be optimised. The case data underline the fact that very few children will ever conform to the hypothetical plan and the clinician will be required to mediate between the therapeutic philosophy and the child.

The alterations to the plan described above were the result of the clinical judgement of the therapist. They have been analysed retrospectively in an attempt to explicate the reasoning behind the clinical decision making process. Whilst, initially, this adjustment of the emphasis of the sessions was made solely on the basis of professional judgement, the case studies now completed suggest that there may be grounds for predicting the course of the progression through therapy from the child's response during the early sessions.

However, until evidence can be gathered from a large body of children who have undergone such a remediation programme no predictions can be made nor guidelines specified in advance. The therapy plan must be determined by the judgement of an experienced clinician. These guidelines about the course of therapy are therefore presented tentatively in the hope that the evidence gathered during the research studies will be of use to the clinician in planning and evaluating therapy.

Activities

It could be said that the message of this book has been look after the theory and the practice will take care of itself. Innovative clinicians will find many ways in which to put the principles of Metaphon therapy into practice, ways which will be determined by the characteristics of both the child and the therapist. The logical conclusion to this line of reasoning would be to consider it superfluous to present concrete suggestions for therapy activities. Indeed this view has its attractions considering the excellent quality of the clinicians who have attended Metaphon courses over the past few years. During the workshops on these courses, clinicians have provided ample evidence of being able to convert theory to practice in imaginative ways.

However, there is perhaps another reason for discussing practical issues. Consideration of actual activities can sometimes give more meaning to abstract ideas allowing readers to understand the authors' thesis more fully. Presentation of 'tried and tested' ideas also allows further illustration of the argument that there are as many ways to put the Metaphon philosophy into action as there are children in clinics. To this end the activities described below have been divided into several different groups to try to underline the way in which an individual child's needs and preferences can be taken into account.

The suggestions are presented for several processes divided according to the type of activity: classifying, matching, manipulating, drawing. Whilst drawing is generally a tabletop activity, many of the other games can be played either sitting or moving about depending on the needs and interest of the child.

The activities given here represent those used by the authors with pre-school children. However, it is a fairly simple conversion to translate many of the games so that they are applicable to young school age children. The referent pictures can be replaced or supplemented by graphemes as appropriate.

SYSTEMIC SIMPLIFYING PROCESSES

FRICATION/STOPPING

1. *Classifying: objects* – straws, snakes, sausages; *sounds* – sound making toys, musical instruments; *phonemes*.

2. *Matching: referent pictures* – e.g. Mr Long and Mr Short ; *objects* – straws, bananas, roads; *sounds/phonemes*.
3. *Drawing:* long/short snakes, socks on washing line, sausages, flowers in vases with long/short stems.
4. *Manipulating objects:* putting l/s scarves on snowmen; building l/s towers of bricks; moving something up l/s ladders; playing dominoes with l/s cards; putting l/s objects (fruit, flowers, leaves) on a tree; putting l/s flowers in vases; feeding l/s objects (bananas, sausages) to a bird/puppet; adding l/s hair to faces/heads; sticking l/s snakes in the grass; making l/s streamers; making a l/s race track.

FRONTING/BACKING

1. *Classifying: objects/pictures* – front/back of people, toys, houses, trains, buses; *phonemes*.
2. *Matching: referent pictures* – e.g. Mr Front/Mr Back pictorial representations; *objects* – trucks, trains, chairs, blackboard, people; *actions* – running to front/back of objects.
3. *Drawing:* parts on front/back of house, person, train, truck; making a mark under a referent picture; drawing people or objects at front/back of a house, bus or train.
4. *Manipulating objects:* feeding puppet at front/back of mouth; posting letters at front/back of house; putting pictures or stars on front/back of drawings, objects, people; moving something up ladders at front/back of houses, Mr Front's/Mr Back's ladder; sitting/putting doll at front/back of objects, table, blackboard, house, bus; making a track at the front/back of a table.

VOICING

1. *Classifying: sounds* – sound making toys, musical instruments; *actions* – walking like Mr Noisy/Mr Whisper; *phonemes*.
2. *Matching: referent pictures* – e.g. Mr Noisy/Mr Whisper; *sounds/phonemes*.
3. *Drawing:* objects that make noisy/quiet sounds; putting a mark/tick under a relevant picture.
4. *Manipulating:* posting letters in Mr N/Mr W's letter box; building a pile of bricks on a referent picture; putting stars on appropriate quiet and noisy pictures, baby sleeping/crying; making a quiet vehicle (a bike) or a noisy vehicle (a lorry or truck) move along a track.

LIQUID GLIDING

1. *Classifying: sounds* according to whether they are 'happy/friendly' etc. (Mr Happy/Friendly sings la, la) or grumpy (Mr Grumpy growls

rrrr) or scary (Mr Scary goes wooo); *people/pictures/animals/ phonemes* (as to whether they are happy/grumpy/scary).

2. *Matching: referent pictures; actions, sounds, phonemes.*
3. *Drawing:* animals in e.g. Mr Grumpy/Scary's cage; making a mark/tick under referent picture.
4. *Manipulating:* feeding Mr Happy/Grumpy etc. puppets with sausages; building a tower on appropriate referent pictures; posting letters in e.g. Mr Happy/Scary's letter boxes; moving referent pictures along a race track.

STRUCTURAL SIMPLIFYING PROCESSES

INITIAL CONSONANT DELETION

1. *Classifying: objects* – animals with/without heads, trains with/without engines, carts with/without horses; *syllables* – as to whether they have e.g. 'engine sounds' or not.
2. *Matching: referent pictures/objects/syllables.*
3. *Drawing:* animals with/without heads, trains with/without engines, trucks with/without cabs.
4. *Manipulating:* pull apart animal toys; completing animal jigsaws; putting a star under one of a pair of referent pictures; moving trains with/without engines around a track.

FINAL CONSONANT DELETION

1. *Classifying: objects* – animals with/without tails, trains with/without carriages/guards vans, horses with/without carts; *syllables* – as to whether they have e.g. tail sounds or not.
2. *Matching: referent pictures/objects/syllables.*
3. *Drawing:* animals with/without tails, animals with silly tails, trains with/without carriages/guards vans, lorries or trucks with/without trailers.
4. *Manipulating:* pull apart animal toys; completing animal jigsaws; building trains with/without carriages; putting a star under one of a pair of referent pictures; moving engines with/without carriages around a track.

CLUSTER REDUCTION

1. *Classifying: objects* – carts with one or two horses, trains with one or two engines, monsters with one or two heads; *sounds* – contrasting two notes on a musical instrument with three; *syllables.*
2. *Matching: referent pictures/objects/syllables.*
3. *Drawing:* carts with one or two horses, trains with one or two engines, monsters with one or two heads, putting a tick/mark under

the relevant picture, drawing heads with one or two hats.

4. *Manipulating:* moving trains with two engines, carts with two horses round track; building towers on referent pictures; putting on one or two hats; building lines of two or three bricks; building queues of two or three people.

In many cases the activities given in these examples will be most applicable during Phase 1 of therapy when the child is exploring the properties of sounds and the sound system. At Phase 1 Word Level the clinician will need to find minimal pair items which represent the contrast the child is collapsing. Examples of minimal pairs which can be pictorially represented can be found in the Metaphon Resource Pack (Dean et al., 1990).

During Phase 2 Word Level the clinician can set the core activity (see Chapter 6) within any game the child wishes to play. Board games may be useful at this stage so that the child's attention is not diverted by any gross motor activity. The child and clinician alternate turns at the core activity with turns at the accompanying game.

When the child reaches Phase 2 Sentence Level the activity will generally revolve around the sentence in which the minimal pair is placed. The following sentences have been found to be useful and adaptable contexts:

Run and jump on ___
Go and sit on the ___
Can you find the ___?
Can you stick the star/banana under the ___?
Post the ___
Put a tick under the ___
Put a brick on the ___
Jump over the ___
Fish for the ___
Give mummy the ___
Can you see the ___?
Put the ___ in the (bucket/box/sandpit)
Can you hide the ___ under the table/in the bin/in the sandpit/under your chair?
Post the ___ in the letter box
Stick the ___ on the board
Hang the ___ on the washing line
Jump into the ___ island
Draw a ___ in the garden

Can you give me/mummy the ___ and the ___?
Can you put a cross under the ___ and the ___?
Find the ___ and the ___

Pull out a ___ and a ___ from the bucket
Jump over the ___ and the ___

These contexts are grouped to illustrate the way that they can be manipulated depending upon the child's needs. The final set of sentence contexts require the child and clinician to incorporate two items from a choice of, probably, four minimal pair items such as tea/key/tar/car. This obviously increases the complexity of the task as do sentences or activities which put an increased memory loading upon the child. The clinician must be aware of all these factors when selecting the sentence contexts.

To illustrate how the activities above can be used within the hypothetical therapy plan presented earlier in the chapter we will now give two examples of notional intervention programmes (Tables 4 and 5)

Table 4 Notional therapy plan for targeting stopping of fricatives

Session	Therapy level	Activity
	Phase 1	
1	Concept/Sound Level	Feed long/short sausages to l/s snakes
	Concept/Sound Level	Draw l/s socks on a washing line
	Phoneme Level*	Blow cotton wool balls with l/s straws
2	Concept/Sound Level	Successful game from Session 1
	Phoneme Level*	Draw/stick l/s snakes in the grass
	Phoneme Level	Move Mr L/Mr S up l/s ladders
3	Phoneme Level	Draw l/s hair on heads
	Word Level*	Build towers of bricks on Mr L/S
	Word Level*	Successful game from previous sessions
4	Phoneme Level	Drawing l/s flowers in vases
	Word Level*	Successful game from previous sessions
	Word Level*	Putting a star under pictures of Mr L/S
	Phase 1 and 2	
5	Word Level* (Phase 1)	Successful game from previous sessions
	Word Level (Phase 2)	Appropriate chosen game
	Word Level (Phase 2)	Appropriate chosen game
6	Word Level* (Phase 1)	Successful game from previous sessions
	Word Level (Phase 2)	Appropriate chosen game
	Word Level (Phase 2)	Appropriate chosen game
	Phase 2	
7	Word Level	Appropriate chosen game
	Sentence Level	Put the ___ in the bucket
	Sentence Level	Go and sit on the ___
8	Sentence Level	Find ___ in the sandpit/box
	Sentence Level	Stick ___ and ___ on the board
	Sentence Level	Put one foot on ___ and one on ___

*Therapist only speaker

both aimed at eliminating systemic simplifying processes. To try to simulate actual events in therapy it is suggested that the child may wish to 'replay' activities that have been enjoyed in previous sessions. During Phase 2 Word Level the clinician is free to choose any game that the child enjoys.

It cannot be stressed too strongly that these plans are merely notional illustrations designed to give the clinician a clearer picture of the way that the concepts underlying the Metaphon approach can be translated into practice. We are always hearing, with great interest, of the many imaginative ways in which therapists have applied the Metaphon philosophy to their management of children with phonological disorders.

Table 5 Notional therapy plan for targeting fronting process

Session	Therapy level	Activity
	Phase 1	
1	Concept/Sound Level	Put dolls at front/back of a train/bus
	Concept/Sound Level	Draw body parts/clothes on Mr F/B
	Phoneme Level*	Feed puppet at f/b of mouth
2	Concept/Sound Level	Successful game from Session 1
	Phoneme Level*	Post letters at f/b of a house.
	Phoneme Level	Stick stars on f/b of a picture of a train
3	Phoneme Level	Draw hair on f/b of heads.
	Word Level	Build towers of bricks on Mr F/B
	Word Level	Successful game from previous sessions
4	Phoneme Level	Drawing food at f/b of an animal's mouth
	Word Level*	Successful game from previous session
	Word Level*	Putting a star under pictures of Mr F/B
	Phase 1 and 2	
5	Word Level* (Phase 1)	Successful game from previous sessions
	Word Level (Phase 2)	Appropriate chosen game
	Word Level (Phase 2)	Appropriate chosen game
6	Word Level* (Phase 1)	Successful game from previous sessions
	Word Level (Phase 2)	Appropriate chosen game
	Word Level (Phase 2)	Appropriate chosen game
	Phase 2	
7	Word Level	Appropriate chosen game
	Sentence Level	Put the ___ in the bucket
	Sentence Level	Go and sit on the ___
8	Sentence Level	Find ___ in the sandpit/box
	Sentence Level	Stick ___ and ___ on the board
	Sentence Level	Put one foot on ___ and one on ___

*Therapist only speaker

Having looked at hypothetical therapy plans we will now turn to some real life clinical sessions using three of the children described in detail in Chapter 3. We will look at each child week by week, list the Metaphon Phase and Level for the week, the aims of each session, the activities that were used and the therapist's evaluation. We have, as far as possible, reproduced this information directly from the case notes, occasionally making some very small grammatical changes to avoid potential misunderstanding.

Jack

Process: Syllable Initial Voicing of Plosives

Session 1

Metaphon Level: Phase 1 Concept and Phoneme Levels

Aims

1. To introduce the concepts of 'quiet', or 'whispered', and 'noisy'.
2. To introduce pictures of 'Mr Quiet/Whisper' and 'Mr Noisy' and encourage use of these labels.
3. To introduce quiet /whisper and noisy non-speech sounds and encourage awareness that sounds can vary along this dimension.

Tasks

1. Introduce 'Mr Whisper/Mr Noisy' puppets. Therapist will make voiceless/voiced sounds and Jack is to determine which puppet would make each sound.
2. Therapist will show Jack 'Mr Whisper/Mr Noisy' referent cards. Jack is to make an appropriate response on musical instruments.
3. Introduce 'Mr Whisper/Mr Noisy' speech sounds and talk about concepts of whispered and noisy as applied to speech sounds. Jack to respond by putting a mark under pictures of 'Mr Whisper/Mr Noisy' on the blackboard.

Evaluation

Jack was a little slow to use the labels of 'Mr Whisper/Mr Noisy', although he understood the concept, so a lot of time was spent talking about using these words (i.e. what the puppets and pictures were called).

Session 2

Metaphon Level: Phase 1 Concept, Phoneme and Word Levels

Aims

1. To make sure Jack understands the concepts of whisper and noisy and that his use of the terminology is appropriate and consistent.
2. To introduce the idea that phonemes vary along the dimensions of whisper/noisy and encourage Jack to reflect on his own sound system.
3. To introduce the concept that words contain whisper and noisy sounds.

Tasks

1. To check understanding of concept, draw 'Mr Whisper /Noisy' referent cards out of a container and match to pictures of musical instruments.
2. Jack to draw 'Mr Whisper /Noisy'. Therapist will produce a range of voiced and voiceless fricatives and stops. Jack to respond by putting a mark under appropriate picture.
3. Therapist will produce a range of phonemes and Jack to respond by putting 'Mr Whisper/Mr Noisy' on pictures of a bicycle (whisper) and a van (noisy).
4. Introduce minimal pairs of 'pea/bee'.

Evaluation

Jack's use of the labels was accurate and consistent and recognition of phonemes was also usually accurate. At the beginning of the session the therapist made a large distinction in intensity between the voiced and voiceless sounds and gradually reduced this over time. Jack's recognition of fricatives at Phoneme Level was always accurate. When words were introduced he said [piz] when looking at the pea and then after the activity said that there were [biz] (peas) and [biz] (bees) on the cards. He was inconsistent in recognition of the therapist's production of voice/voiceless sounds at Word Level.

Session 3

Metaphon Level: Phase 1 Concept, Phoneme and Word Levels

Aims

As in session 2.

Tasks

1. Therapist and Jack to act as speakers and produce a range of

phonemes, supported by referent cards. Listener to respond by carrying out an action in the same way as 'Mr Whisper/Mr Noisy'.
2. Therapist to present 'pea/bee'. Jack to put pictures of pea/bee on top of a baby sleeping (whisper) or a vacuum cleaner (noisy).
3. Therapist to present 'toe/dough'. Jack to make appropriate 'Mr Whisper/ Mr Noisy' puppet say or do something.

Evaluation

Consistent recognition of concept in phonemes. Frequently consistent at Word Level. Jack was seen to be actively reflecting on the quality of the sounds and on a number of occasions changed his mind about which dimension was represented. Therapist attempted to keep the same intensity at both Word and Phoneme Level. Jack produced voiceless stops appropriately at times, and sometimes spontaneously in discussion in 'pea' and 'toe'. A period of active reflection on the nature of the sounds produced by the therapist appeared to be required before Jack could achieve consistent production.

Session 4

Metaphon Level: Phase 1 Concept, Phoneme and Word Levels

Aims

As in session 2 with the addition of:
4. To encourage Jack to produce a range of 'noisy/whisper' phonemes using referent cards.

Tasks

1. Jack and therapist to take it in turns to produce a range of 'whisper/noisy' sounds; listener to respond by shaking appropriate shaker.
2. Therapist presents 'pin/bin'. Jack to respond by putting a star under a picture of a drum (noisy) or a triangle (whisper).
3. Therapist presents 'coat/goat'. Response is to run a bike or a van along a track.

Evaluation

Jack's recognition of phonemes was always accurate. His production of phoneme was restricted to producing /p/ and /t/ for whisper and /d/ for noisy despite the therapist providing many alternative examples. Jack was always accurate in recognition of 'pin/bin' but sometimes had difficulty with 'coat/goat' (task 3) but his concentration had waned by this time. It was necessary to work on this more before moving to Phase 2.

Session 5

Metaphon Level: Phase 1 Word Level and Phase 2 Word Level

Aims

As in session 4 with the addition of:
5. Phase 2 activities to make Jack aware of the message conveying capacity of words and that a change in dimension of whisper/noisy leads to a change in meaning.

Tasks

1. For Phase 1 Word Level, therapist to present 'coat/goat' and 'Kate/gate'. Jack to respond by running bike or van along a track.
2. For Phase 2, therapist and Jack to take it in turns to be speaker and listener to pass 'toe/dough' secret messages. Fuzzy felt game to accompany.
3. Phase 2. Minimal pair: 'bin/pin'.
4. Phase 2. Minimal pair: 'pea/bee'.

Evaluation

At Phase 1 Jack was quite consistent in recognition and produced /b;d/ for noisy and /p;t/ for whisper sounds. In task 2 (Phase 2 Word Level) Jack produced voice/voiceless contrast accurately on all but one occasion, but it was noted that there was no carryover to connected speech. Jack was unreflective and impulsive in response to this task and the therapist questioned whether he had grasped the central concept although he was successful in making distinctions.

Session 6

Metaphon Level: Phase 1 Word Level and Phase 2 Sentence Level

Aims

As in session 5.

Tasks

1. Phase 2. Minimal pair: 'toe/dough'.

2. Phase 2. Minimal pair: 'Kate /gate'. Jack to respond by putting a star on the drum or the triangle.
3. Phase 2 Sentence Level: 'Run and jump on the pea/bee'.
4. Phase 2 Sentence Level: 'Put the toe/dough in the bucket'.

Evaluation

At Phase 1 Word Level there was consistent recognition. At Phase 2 Sentence Level in task 3 there was some success as speaker but this was not consistent. Task 4 resulted in much more consistent success. If the therapist asked him to repeat when she had not understood he simply made his voice louder at first. However, towards the end of the session he appeared to become much more aware of listener confusion and corrected voiced to voiceless when required. Jack appeared to be very much a 'listener blamer'.

Session 7

Metaphon Level: Phase 1 Word Level and Phase 2 Sentence Level

Aims

As in session 5.

Tasks

1. Phase 1 Word Level: Presentation of 'coat/goat' and 'pin/bin'. Jack to respond by blowing an appropriate sound on a recorder. Jack also to be encouraged to produce a range of 'whisper/noisy' phonemes during this activity.
2. Phase 2 Sentence Level: 'Go and find the pin/bin in the sandpit'.
3. Phase 2 Sentence Level: 'Go and stick the coat/goat on the board'.

Evaluation

For Phase 1 activities, recognition was good, but there was no increase in the range of whisper/noisy sounds produced by Jack. Task 2 resulted in adult-like distinctions. Response in task 3 was very interesting; Jack was obviously very aware of the need to change the dimension of the sound in order to convey his message. He underwent metalinguistic repair before giving the correct message, not on the instance of listener confusion. For example, he said a number of times 'Go and stick the goat, no not that one the coat', before the therapist could carry out the activity. It was apparent that he was reflecting, quite consciously, on the effect that his change of dimension was having on the message.

Session 8

Metaphon Level: Phase 1 Word Level and Phase 2 Sentence Level

Aims
As in session 5.

Tasks

1. Phase 1 Word Level: therapist to present 'Kate/gate' and 'pea/bee'. Jack to respond by putting a star under a picture of a vacuum cleaner (noisy) or a dog sleeping (whisper). Jack also to take role of speaker.
2. Phase 2 Sentence Level: 'Can you hide the Kate/gate then/coat/goat under the table?'
3. Phase 2 Sentence Level: 'Go and sit on the pin/bin'.

Evaluation

There were no difficulties with Phase 1 activities. Consistent adult like distinctions between 'pin/bin' were made. The velar distinctions were more difficult and were accompanied by a more conscious awareness that a change of dimension was necessary. There were instances of listener blamer, but Jack was more prepared to understand that if the listener responded in a different manner to that expected then he had to modify his utterance to correspond.

Summary

Session 8 marked the end of treatment for syllable initial voicing. Monitoring trials revealed 0% occurrence of the process and a considerable decrease in some other processes. An interesting feature of Jack's treatment in terms of therapy planning is that relatively little time was spent at Phase 2 Word Level and rather more at Phase 2 Sentence Level. The reason for this appeared to be that, although Jack had no difficulty in making distinctions between minimal pairs, there was little carryover initially into connected speech and he appeared to make little if any connection between the therapy tasks and communication. The therapist described him as an unreflective child in the early stages of therapy, but the strategy of spending time at Phase 2 Sentence Level appears not only to have helped to establish the voice/voiceless contrast in connected speech but also to have had this effect through an increase in reflection and self-monitoring as illustrated by Jack's self-correction noted during session 7.

Therapy for stopping of fricatives was started in the following session. Jack had six sessions working on this process. Progress was excellent with once again quick resolution of the simplifying process. We saw in Chapter 3 that Jack had no further therapy after this and that when reviewed, a year after starting therapy, he had very few phonological problems. Six months later when he was reviewed again he had only intermittent fronting of /θ/ and was discharged.

Barry

Process: Velar Fronting (Syllable Initial)

Session 1

Metaphon Level: Phase 1 Concept and Phoneme Level

Aims

1. To introduce concept of front and back.
2. To use referents of 'Mr Front and Mr Back' and encourage use of these terms.
3. To introduce the metalinguistic concept of front and back as applied to tongue position in mouth.

Tasks

1. To decide which was the front/back of a train and Barry to put an object on front/back as requested.
2. Therapist to introduce pictures of 'Mr Front' and 'Mr Back' as she sits on front/back of train. Role reversal with Barry sitting on appropriate part of train in response to pictures.
3. Therapist to introduce alveolar and velar phonemes showing appropriate picture of 'Mr Front/Mr Back' and Barry to stick stars on front/back of pictured train.

Evaluation

Barry understood the concept of front/back very well and used the labels consistently himself. Whilst the therapist was talking about the phonemes he was attempting to make velars when she did and was quite consistent at recognising alveolars and velars.

Session 2

Metaphon Level: Phase 1 Phoneme and Word Level

Aims

1. To check that Barry can use labels consistently.

2. To indicate to Barry that speech sounds can be classified on the front/back dimension and to make him aware that he can manipulate sounds on this dimension.
3. To indicate to Barry that words also contain front/back sounds and that they signal change in meaning.

Tasks

1. Therapist to produce a range of front/back phonemes and Barry to respond by putting a mark under picture of 'Mr Front/Mr Back'.
2. Therapist to produce a range of front/back phonemes and Barry to respond by feeding a puppet a banana at the front/back of its mouth.
3. Therapist to present the words 'dough' and 'go' and Barry to respond by drawing objects on the front and back of the picture of a house.

Evaluation

Barry was reasonably consistent in labelling sounds correctly; /k/ and /g/ were always correct but sometimes he also said that /t/ and /d/ were back sounds. On a few occasions he produced /g/ when the therapist did and once he produced it spontaneously. He was very aware that he could manipulate sounds on the front/back dimension and visibly attemped to move his tongue around his mouth. He also showed reasonable consistency in recognising front/back dimension in words.

Session 3

Aims

As for session 2.

Tasks

1. Therapist and Barry to take turns to produce a range of front/back sounds. Response to add parts to front and back of drawing of a man.
2 Therapist to present 'tar/car' with referent. Barry to respond by pinning picture on to front/back of blackboard.
3. Therapist to present 'tap/cap' with referent. Response to post letters through front/back letter box of a house.

Evaluation

Barry's mother reported that he had spontaneously produced

'go/dough' when using the words in a front/back recognition activity. In therapy Barry produced only /t/ and /k/ in relation to referents at Phoneme Level activity but produced /g/ once on prompting. The 'tar/car' minimal pair prompted spontaneous production of correct 'car' and a correct response to the therapist asking 'what was the front/back sound in that word?' He had no difficulty in recognising 'tap/cap' distinctions by the therapist, but when he attempted to say 'cap' he was very confused and when asked what the back sound was in 'cap' he replied by saying 'tap' or [t]. Confusion lessened towards the end of the session.

There was no therapy in the following week because Barry had a hearing test but his mother reported that he had initiated activities where he said a word and she had to say whether it had a front or back sound in it.

Session 4:

Metaphon Level: Phase 1 Phoneme and Word Levels, Phase 2 Word Level

Aims

1. To encourage Barry to reflect on the front/back dimension of phonemes.
2. To encourage him to produce a range of front/back phonemes using referent.
3. To convey to Barry the importance, and knowledge, of the message conveying capacity of words and the ability to initiate repair in the case of listener confusion.

Tasks

1 Take turns to produce range of front/back sounds. Response to stick snakes in grass drawn on the front and back of the blackboard.
2. Phase 2 Word Level: minimal pair 'cap/tap', accompanying lotto game.
3. Phase 2 Word Level: minimal pair 'day/gay', accompanying fuzzy felt game.

Evaluation

Phase 1 activity showed evidence of easy production of front/back sounds, with consistent awareness and reflection. The same awareness was present during the Phase 2 activities with consistent production of correct minimal pair.

Session 5

Metaphon Level: Phase 1 Word Level, Phase 2 Word and Sentence Levels

Aims

As for session 4.

Tasks

1. Phoneme Level: listener to respond by putting card in front/back of a house.
2. Phase 2 Word Level: minimal pairs (four words presented in single activity), 'tea/key/tar/car'. Accompanying game, fuzzy felt or lotto.
3. Phase 2 Sentence Level: 'Put the dough/go in the bucket'.

Evaluation

Phase 1 work was accurate and Barry could achieve adult contrast at both Word and Sentence Level during Phase 2 work. There were some good examples of repair during this session in response to listener confusion. This was particularly apparent when an incorrect response was commented on, for example ' Do you think you should have the one with the back sound there?'

Session 6

Metaphon Level: Phase 1 Word and Phase 2 Sentence Level

Aims

As for session 5.

Tasks

1. Therapist produces 'dough/go' and 'day/Gay'. Barry to respond by sticking a star on the front/back of a train.
2. Phase 2 Sentence Level: 'Run and jump on the tap/cap/tar/car'.
3. Phase 2 Sentence Level: 'Find the tea/key in the sandpit'.

Evaluation

Barry's mother reported that Barry seemed a 'little fed up' with the activities. The therapist observed that this was reflected in his response to Phase 1 activities during therapy, where he gave inconsistent responses. However, Phase 2 activities were well done, but Barry insisted on inserting 'Go' at the start of the direction when he was speaker and this was produced as [do]. On two occasions the therapist brought his attention to this and he repaired spontaneously, but there was little carryover into connected speech outside the therapy tasks.

Session 7

Metaphon Level: Phase 1 Word Level and Phase 2 Sentence Level

Aims

As for session 6.

Tasks

1. Phase 1 Word Level: 'tea/key/tar/car' words used. Response to stick a banana on the front/back of a tree.
2. Phase 2 Sentence Level: 'Put the dough/go', or 'day/Gay, under the table'.
3. Phase 2 Sentence Level: 'Go over and stand on the tap/cap/tar/car'.

Evaluation

Once again Barry gave the impression of being slightly bored with the activities. There was still little evidence of carryover into connected speech outside the therapy tasks and he did not always repair immediately. Tasks were well done and 'go' was always used accurately in task 2, but in task 3 it would only be accurate at the start of a sentence which contained another velar.

It was decided to discontinue working on this process for this day.

Conclusions and Comments

Barry responded well to working on this process and made rapid progress. He appeared to have no difficulty in making distinctions between alveolar and velar phonemes in therapy tasks, and gave good evidence of reflection. However, the therapist was concerned at the apparently slow rate of generalisation into connected speech. We would argue that this gradual pattern of change is in line with the Hewlett model (Chapter 2) and that it takes time for a new motor plan to replace an habitual one.

Our confidence that change would come about was confirmed by Barry's subsequent progress. The therapist went on to target initial consonant deletion, for 12 sessions. Barry found this process much more difficult to eradicate and there were periods during this stage of therapy when he was reluctant to come to clinic. A breakthrough appeared to come at the seventh session of working on this process when the therapist started her evaluation with the comment 'a wonderful session'. She then went on to describe how Barry started to be able to discover how to make distinctions between a vowel and a word consisting of fricative + vowel, for example /i/ and 'sea', in a series of gradual stages. From then on progress was rapid. Therapy was discontinued after treating these two processes. When reviewed 7 months later his only remaining simplifying process was /θ/ → /f/. He was therefore discharged.

Jamie

Process 1: Initial Consonant Deletion (all voiceless phonemes)

Session 1

Metaphon Level: Phase 1 Concept and Syllable Level

Aims

1 To discover whether Jamie is aware of the concept 'beginning' or 'start' and is able to use this terminology.
2. To introduce non-meaningful syllables and show Jamie that words may, or may not, have a consonant at the beginning.

Tasks

1. To talk to Jamie about animals, trains etc., as having something at the beginning.
2. To ask Jamie to draw something with a beginning.
3. To introduce non-meaningful syllables and ask Jamie whether he can hear an 'engine sound' (consonant) at the beginning or not.

Evaluation

Jamie was very aware of the concepts of 'beginning' and 'start' and was quick to start using them. In task 3 he was usually able to recognise whether the syllables did or did not have an engine sound at the start.

Session 2

Metaphon Level: Phase 1 Syllable and Word Level

Aims

1. To check that Jamie is aware of and can use the concept of beginning to apply to words.
2. To show Jamie that we can manipulate the property of beginning to produce two different words.
3. To encourage him to reflect on this property and to encourage him to attempt to manipulate it himself.

Tasks

1. Therapist to present non-meaningful syllables. Jamie to respond by adding on/taking off heads of plastic animals.
2. Therapist to present 'ee/sea'. Response to put together or pull apart front parts of jigsaws.
3. Therapist to present 'oo/two'. Jamie to respond by drawing trains with or without engines.

Evaluation

Jamie was very quick to recognise the concept as it applied to words and was consistent in his recognition of them. During discussion the therapist twice exaggerated the first sound, for example 't..t..t..two'; Jamie responded by saying [ku] (he backed alveolars to velars). He was a very reflective child.

Session 3

Metaphon Level: Phase 1 Syllable and Word Level

Aims

As for session 2, plus
4. To encourage Jamie to produce a range of V or CV syllables.

Tasks

1. Jamie and therapist to take turns to be speaker and listener and produce non-meaningful syllables in response to a referent (trains with/without engines). Listener to respond by putting heads on, or leaving off, animal jigsaws.
2. Therapist presents 'chair/air'. Response taking off, or putting on, heads of plastic animals.
3. Therapist to present 'arm/farm'. Response putting trains together or leaving them apart.

Evaluation

Jamie was unsure about what nonsense syllables to produce, although he did produce [fa] as CV and /i/ as a V syllable. He always recognised syllables appropriately and had no difficulties with relating appropriate concepts to the minimal pair words. Twice he attempted to say the words after the therapist and was able to include some kind of consonant.

Session 4

Metaphon Level: Phase 1 Syllable and Word Level

Aims

As for last week.

Tasks

1. Therapist and Jamie to take it in turns to present non-meaningful syllables. Response plastic animals and heads.
2. Therapist to present 'ee/key'. Response to draw lorries with/without cabs at petrol station.
3. Therapist to present 'oo/shoe'. Response to join jigsaws together or not.

Evaluation

This was a very reflective session. Jamie was very interested in words that had initial consonants and was particularly interested in /f/, so during the course of the session he pointed out lots of words beginning with /f/. During task 1 he was a little slow to think of words with engine sounds usually producing [fa] or [fi]. He was usually successful in tasks 2 and 3 although he would sometimes say there was an engine sound when there was not.

Session 5

Metaphon Level: Phase 1 Syllable and Word Level, Phase 2 Word Level

Aims

As for last week, with the addition of:
5. Indicate to Jamie that he can manipulate the syllable structure to create word meaning distinctions.

6. Encourage repair if the listener is confused.

Tasks

1. Therapist and child to take it in turns to make up non-meaningful syllables.
2. Phase 2 Word Level: minimal pair, 'ee/sea'.
3. Phase 2 Word Level: minimal pair, 'oo/two'.
4. Phase 2 Word Level: minimal pair, 'air/chair'.

Evaluation

Jamie was very receptive to stimulation to encourage change. He was very aware that engine sounds were necessary if he was to be fully understood. Even in his conversation he was making lots of attempts at including word initial voiceless consonants, and was even using /t/ rather than /k/ at times. During tasks he always created a distinction on his first attempt.

Session 6

Metaphon Level: Phase 2 Word Level and Sentence Level

Aims

As last session.

Tasks

1. Phase 2 Word Level: minimal pair 'ee/key'.
2. Phase 2 Sentence Level: 'Run and jump on the oo/shoe'.
3. Phase 2 Sentence Level: 'Put the ee/sea in the cup'.

Evaluation

Jamie's mother reported that Jamie said that the two year old son of his child minder was 'forgetting his engine sounds'. Good progress was made in using appropriate words within a sentence and he usually used /k/ at the beginning of 'cup' in task 3. Much more spontaneous use of targets was made in conversation.

Session 7

Metaphon Level: Phase 2 Sentence Level

Aims

As for last week.

Tasks

1. 'Stick the ee/sea/key, and the ee/sea/key on the door'.
2. 'Go and sit on the oo/shoe/two and the oo/shoe/two'.
3. 'Hide the air/chair in the bucket/under the table' etc.

Evaluation

This was another successful session with Jamie spontaneously putting initial fricatives on words other than the target words in the sentences, for example in 'sit ' and 'hide'. He was also making many spontaneous repairs in his conversation and was now very aware of initial fricatives. The monitoring trial revealed 0% occurrence of initial fricative deletion, so work on this process was terminated.

Treatment started on Process 2: Backing

Session 8

Metaphon Level: Phase 1 Concept, Sound and Phoneme Levels

Aims

1. To introduce the concept of 'front/back' and decide if Jamie has knowledge of this concept.
2. To encourage use of these terms.

Tasks

1. To sit on the front/back of a train constructed from chairs.
2. Show train referent cards with flags at the front/back of the train and ask Jamie to sit on appropriate seat on front/back of train.
3. Introduce 'Mr Front' and 'Mr Back' and discuss the sort of noises they like.
4. Introduce speech sounds that 'Mr Front' and 'Mr Back' like.

Evaluation

Jamie had no difficulty in understanding the concept of front/back and was quick to use the terms. He was also able to match speech sounds to the concept, but not consistently.

(*Authors' note.* From this session until the end of the therapy period, sessions were given twice, rather than once, weekly because of Jamie's impending move out of the district.)

Session 9

Metaphon Level: Phase 1 Concept, Phoneme and Word Level

Aims

1. To check that Jamie is understanding and using the terms front/back consistently.
2. To introduce Jamie to the fact that speech sounds can be classified as front/back and encourage reflection on this contrast.
3. To encourage Jamie to listen for sounds in words.

Tasks

1. Therapist to present as front sounds – /p,b,t,d,f,v/ and back sounds as – /s,z, ʃ, k, g/. Jamie to respond by feeding a bird puppet at front or back of its mouth.

   (*Authors' note:* The inclusion of fricatives and the application of the front/back dimension in this way was an attempt to encourage Jamie to use the alveolar place of articulation. In effect an attempt was being made to treat the backing of alveolar stops and fronting of fricatives at the same time, probably because of his impending departure.)

2. Therapist to present 'bite/bike'. Jamie to respond by putting hair on front/back of a head.
3. Therapist to present 'rough/rush'. Jamie to respond by putting a star on the front/back of a picture of a train.

Evaluation

Classification of these sounds was quite difficult for Jamie. He was able to classify /k/ and /g/ as back and /p,b/ and /f/ as front sounds, but the other sounds were not consistently classified. He had no difficulty in recognising what sounds were being represented in the minimal pair words. He was also able to tell the therapist that 'rush' had /ʃ/ in it, but also asked where the 'engine sound' was as well.

Session 10

Metaphon Level: Phase 1 Phoneme and Word Levels

Aims

As for last week with the addition of:
3. To encourage Jamie to tell the therapist front and back sounds.

Tasks

1. Therapist and Jamie to take turns at telling each other front/back sounds. Response is to stick stars on the front/back of a train picture.
2. Therapis to present 'tea/key', 'mud/mug'. Jamie to put stickers on the front/back of a person.
3. Therapist to present 'nice/knife'; same response as above from Jamie.

Evaluation

Jamie was not very forthcoming in terms of sounds and was really only able to give /p/ as a front sound and /ʃ/ as a back sound with any consistency. He was able to identify front/back sounds in activity 2 but had some difficulty with activity 3. He attempted to use /t/ and /d/ as front sounds when asked for example 'What Mr Front sound did you hear in tea?' but he could not produce these and said /k/ and /g/ instead. He was aware of the fact that he was using the wrong sound and said at one stage 'I can't say that'.

(*Authors' note:* Therapist expressed concern in the notes that she thought that she was moving Jamie on too quickly and that he had no time to reflect on the sounds.)

Session 11

Metaphon Level: Phase 1 Phoneme and Word Levels

Aims

As for last week.

Tasks

1. Jamie and therapist to take it in turns to produce sounds that are front/back. Response is to put snakes in grass at the front/back of a chair.
2. Therapist to present 'bat/back', 'bite/bike'. Response is to post letters in front or back of a post box.
3. Therapist to present 'rough/rush'. Response to stick something on front/back of a cupboard door.

Evaluation

Jamie had begun to use /t/ in conversation, for example, 'tank', 'Thomas' and 'table' and was offering /t/ and sometimes /d/ as front sounds. He was also making some attempts at spontaneous repair, for example changing from /ku/ to /tu/. Jamie was not volunteering /f/, /s/ or /ʃ/ and appeared to be unaware of where /s/ and /ʃ/ fitted into the scheme of things. He said that he kept 'forgetting' them, but had no difficulty in identifying appropriately the sounds the therapist was using in minimal pair words.

Session 12

Metaphon Level: Phase 1 Phoneme Level, Phase 2 Word Level

Aims

1. To encourage Jamie to be aware of the fact that a change of front/back sound will signal and effect a change in meaning.
2. To encourage Jamie to use this awareness to signal the different minimal pair words.
3. To encourage use of metalinguistic repair when the listener is confused.

Tasks

1. Phase 1 Phoneme work.
2. Phase 2 Word Level: 'bat/ back' and, 'bite/bike'.
3. Phase 2 Word Level: 'rough/rush'.
4. Phase 2 Word Level: 'mud/mug'.

Evaluation

Jamie was very aware of the need to create a distinction between the front/back sounds and usually managed to do this on his first attempt at passing his 'secret message' or when the therapist pointed to the 'wrong one' if he made an error. In addition he could always identify the front/back sound he was using. He also made corrections in conversation when the listener said 'pardon' or looked confused.

Session 13

Metaphon Level: Phase 2 Word and Sentence Level

Aims

As for last session.

Tasks

1. Phase 2 Word Level: 'nice/knife'.
2. Phase 2 Sentence Level: 'Put the mud /mug under the table'.
3. Phase 2 Sentence Level: 'Run and jump on the bat/back/ bite/bike'.
4. Phase 2 Sentence Level: 'Stick the rough/rush on the door'.

Evaluation

Jamie was usually able to make changes in output and in the final task was often able to use /d/ rather than /g/ in door. In conversation Jamie often used the appropriate front/back sounds spontaneously and was always able to repair in response to listener confusion, or prompting. His mother reported that Jamie was making great advances at home in using /t/ and /d/ and was spontaneously repairing. This was Jamie's last Metaphon session.

Summary

Jamie responded well to Metaphon therapy and made rapid progress despite having a very severe phonological difficulty. Both the treated processes were eliminated before our contact with him ceased. There is no doubt that Jamie was a very reflective child who was very interested in speech sounds and we believe that arousing and encouraging this interest contributed to his rapid progress. We have reported the treatment of the two processes that were treated, to demonstrate that although Jamie was sometimes confused in therapy, particularly during the treatment of backing, he was making spontaneous repairs in his own speech after three sessions of treatment for this process. The therapist wisely responded to this by rapidly progressing to Phase 2 Sentence Level work even though Jamie was still expressing confusion about the classification of some sounds.

We can suggest two possible explanations for this confusion. In her evaluation of this last session the therapist commented at some length on her frustration at having to push Jamie on too quickly and at the rapid pace of therapy. It is evident from her earlier comments that she felt that Jamie's confusion about front/back sounds reported in her evaluation of sessions 9 and 10 resulted from lack of time for reflection. This view supports our supposition of the nature of the learning process during Metaphon therapy; that the therapy situation provides a facilitating environment to enable children to reflect on speech sounds to bring about their own changes to their own phonological systems. It is also possible that some of Jamie's confusion might have been avoided if the front/back concept had been restricted to the contrast between alveolar and velar plosives, that is /t/, /d/ versus /k/, /g/. At a later stage fronting of /s/, /z/ to /f/, /v/ could have been treated separately. As we saw in Chapter 5 it is important to minimise the cognitive demands of the situation to achieve optimum language learning. It is possible that the categorisation of phonemes the therapist was expecting Jamie to use on this occasion was too complex for him to grasp. Whatever the reason for Jamie's initial confusion during some therapy sessions, we saw from the evaluations of the sessions and the outcomes reported in Chapter 3 that Jamie was resolving his phonological difficulties successfully by the end of his period of treatment.

Jamie's case is a good illustration of the importance of noting the child's responses to therapy, and adjusting aims and activities to accommodate these responses to maximise the effectiveness of treatment. Our detailed reporting of the therapy given to these three children and their responses to it illustrates the way in which each step of Metaphon therapy is decided by the child's response in the previous session resulting in the gradual elimination of simplifying processes. These case reports therefore provide a fitting end to this chapter by bringing together the organisation of therapy sessions and the practical activities we discussed earlier in the chapter whilst at the same illustrating the importance of basing therapeutic decisions on the child's response.

Chapter 8
Does Metaphon Therapy Work?

Introduction

In this chapter we discuss in detail the first study we carried out to find out whether Metaphon is an effective treatment method for phonological disorder. We follow this with a brief description of a second efficacy study which we are currently undertaking. The first investigation gave us some very encouraging results but it left some issues unresolved and also raised other very interesting issues. The second, much larger investigation has been designed to address these issues.

Our clinical experience, and that of colleagues and students who had attended our courses, provided general support for our belief that Metaphon therapy constituted an appropriate approach to the remediation of phonological disorder. However, clinical impressions, although valuable, do not provide sufficient support for a treatment method and we felt it necessary to carry out objective, quantitative investigations.

The First Investigation

The aim of this investigation was not only to discover whether Metaphon was effective but also to study patterns of phonological change and their association with metalinguistic change. To this end the research was designed to answer the following questions:

1. Can the targeted area of linguistic development – the phonological system – be accelerated beyond the level which would be expected due to chronological development?
2. Does Metaphon therapy specifically affect those processes which are targeted in therapy or is its effect more general?
3. Can concomitant changes in linguistic awareness provide evidence about the way in which the intervention programme influences the phonological system?

151

In order to answer these questions we designed the experiment to test the following predictions:

1. There would be a significant change in scores on the phonological assessment.
2. There would be no corresponding change in scores on the vocabulary assessment.
3. There would be a significant change in scores on phoneme segmentation and communicative awareness tasks.
4. There would be no corresponding change in sentence segmentation and sentence structure tasks.

These predictions were based on two hypotheses which follow from questions 1 and 2 above. First, that Metaphon therapy will be effective in accelerating phonological development beyond the linguistic change that might be expected with age (as measured by the vocabulary scores). Second, that the nature of Metaphon therapy is such that it will lead to greater change in metaphonological and metacommunicative awareness than in metasyntactic awareness.

Method

Subjects

Thirteen children participated in the investigation, three girls and nine boys. At the start of the study, the children were aged between 3;7 and 4;7 with an average age of 4;1 (ages for each subject can be found in Table 6). The children were referred to the project by local speech therapists working in clinics and nursery schools in the locality of Queen Margaret College, Edinburgh. We obtained parental consent for all the children to participate in the investigation before we started the assessment and treatment programme.

To enable us to exercise some control over possible factors which might selectively influence the outcome of treatment for individual children we used the following criteria when selecting children:

1. The children should not have started school but had to be over the age of 3;6.
   This criterion was used to ensure that the children had not been exposed to formal reading and writing instruction, factors which are known to have an influence on metalinguistic awareness, but would be old enough to participate in this type of therapy.
2. They should present with a problem involving the acquisition of the sound system of their native language, in the absence of known sen-

Table 6 Chronological age (CA), sex, weeks in treatment and number of sessions; all subjects

Subject	CA	Sex	Weeks in treatment	No. of sessions
1	3;7	F	18	16
2	3;8	M	21	15
3	3;8	M	31	20
4	3;8	M	18	14
5	3;8	M	19	18
6	4;0	F	19	13
7	4;1	F	19	17
8	4;1	M	24	20
9	4;2	M	25	19
10	4;4	M	25	18
11	4;4	M	25	19
12	4;5	M	34	25
13	4;7	M	11	13
Range	3;7–4;7		11–34	13–25
Mean	4;1		22.5	17.4

sory, cognitive neurological or physical problems, including hearing impairment.

In other words the children's problems should be specific to the speech sound system and could not be attributed to any known cause.

3. They should be from a monolingual family background.

    This criterion was included as it is known that exposure to more than one language can have a beneficial effect on linguistic awareness.

4. They should have received no previous speech therapy.

    Without this stipulation it would not have been possible to determine whether any observed improvement could be attributed to Metaphon therapy or to some previous intervention procedure.

5. Their comprehension age (as measured on the Reynell Developmental Language Scales (RDLS) (Reynell, 1977)) parenthesis should be no less than 6 months below chronological age.

    A second criterion to determine that the subject's problems are primarily confined to the phonological aspects of language.

6. They should present with at least three phonological processes with occurrence of greater than or equal to 50%.

    This criterion was used to ensure that the subjects were suitable for inclusion in our experimental design.

Design

Because the children involved in the study had all been judged to require, and had been accepted for, speech therapy the design of the investigation was constrained to some extent. We felt we could not, for example, deliberately withhold treatment from any of the children in order to compare the progress of a treated and an untreated group. Our answer to this problem was to design the investigation as a series of single case studies in which each child acted as its own control. This design allows both the study of individual responses to remediation and comparison across the group as a whole (see Code, 1985, and Coltheart, 1989, for examples of single case methodology).

In order to answer the questions posed above the investigation was divided into an assessment phase, a treatment phase and a reassessment phase. We will describe each of the phases in turn.

Assessment Phase

A full phonological assessment using the prototype of The Metaphon Resource Pack (MRP) (Dean et al., 1990), described in Chapter 3, was administered to determine the number and extent of the simplifying processes operating in the child's speech. The British Picture Vocabulary Scales (BPVS) (Dunn et al., 1982) were used to assess vocabulary.

Four tasks, specifically designed for the investigation, to assess different aspects of linguistic awareness were also administered. These were:

1. A phoneme segmentation task to assess phonological awareness. In this task based on Zhurova (1973) the children were asked to segment the initial phoneme of a given word. The task was presented in the form of a game where items of food taken on a picnic were used as the experimental words.
2. A communicative awareness task. This task assessed the children's awareness of the need to make changes to speech output if the listener did not fully understand. Degree of awareness was determined by scoring the children's ability to make changes to their pronunciation of minimal pair words in response to feedback from the experimenter.
3. A sentence structure task. In this task the children were asked to make judgements about the appropriateness of a given sentence by saying whether it was silly or sensible. Some of the sentences were correct and some violated word order rules.
4. A sentence segmentation task. This task was based on a procedure suggested by Fox and Routh (1975) and was designed to test the

children's ability to divide sentences into their constituent words. The task was presented as a game where the children were asked to provide a toy bear with 'just a little bit' of a given sentence to help him to learn to talk.

To determine any potential weaknesses in speech processing ability we also administered auditory discrimination and imitation tasks which were specifically devised for the investigation.

On the basis of the phonological assessment (MRP) three simplifying phonological processes, operating at or near 100%, were selected as the first treated process (Process A), the second treated process (Process B) and the untreated control process (Process C).

Occurrence of each of the three selected processes was measured three times at weekly intervals before treatment started using the Monitoring Procedure from the MRP. Monitoring was repeated every third session during the treatment phase to chart the effect of therapy and repeated again in the reassessment phase.

The MRP monitoring procedure is designed to provide a means of assessing change in the occurrence of one or more phonological processes during a course of therapy. Multiple tokens of single word items, which have not been the focus of therapy, are elicited from the child in a naming task disguised as a colour sorting task. (Full details can be found in Dean et al., 1990.)

Our choice of processes to target for each child was made on clinical criteria. That is we used the type of decision making process described in Chapter 3. This is not an ideal selection procedure for research purposes. It would have been preferable to randomly assign processes to treatment or non-treatment conditions. To some extent this problem was overcome by the fact that over the whole group of subjects different processes could be assigned to different conditions giving some measure of randomness.

Treatment Phase

The subjects were seen weekly for a 30 minute treatment session. Therapy used the procedures of Metaphon therapy as described in Chapters 6 and 7. Treatment was designed so that the intervention (Phase 1 followed by Phase 2) was directed towards Process A until it was operating at approximately 50% occurrence as measured by the relevant monitoring trial. At this point therapy ceased for Process A and was focused on Process B until the end of the treatment phase. Process C was not treated.

We attempted to balance and measure the amount of input provided by the subjects' parents during the treatment phase in the following ways. After assessment, a full explanation of the individual child's phonological difficulties, the rationale behind the treatment and the nature of the therapeutic activities was given in order to provide the same amount of information for all parents. Similarly, the parents were invited to be present during every session. In addition, in an attempt to monitor the amount of practice each child had at home, a worksheet was given each week and parents were asked to record the number of days on which some home practice was undertaken. These worksheets provided information about the concepts being worked on that week and made some general suggestions about how the children could be helped to absorb these concepts.

Reassessment Phase

The following assessments were readministered at the end of the treatment phase:

full phonological assessment (MRP);
vocabulary assessment (BPVS);
the monitoring procedures (MRP);
the four linguistic awareness tasks.

Results

The first task in this section is to record information about the length of treatment and attendance record. Because we were measuring change in an ongoing clinical situation it was not possible to predetermine this. Treatment schedules are influenced by response to therapy and frequency of attendance is dependent upon many factors including parental co-operation, absence for illness and holiday periods. It was therefore inevitable that there would be differences between children in the number of treatment sessions they received, the frequency of their attendance and the total length of time each child was in the treatment phase of the investigation.

The treatment phase lasted on average 22.5 weeks, ranging from 11 to 34 weeks. Of the thirteen subjects, ten attended weekly with occasional brief absences due to sickness or short holidays. Two subjects (3 and 12) were very poor attenders, at times failing to attend for several weeks without making contact. One subject (13) had a short period of twice weekly sessions towards the end of the treatment phase because his family had to move abroad at short notice. Information about the number of sessions and the length of time each child was in the treatment phase can be found in Table 6.

As variables, such as attendance record and length of time in treatment, may influence the outcome of treatment, it is important that these variables are considered and we will return to them below.

Early in this chapter we listed three questions that our investigation set out to answer. We will now take each of these questions in turn and consider the evidence provided by the results of the investigation.

Can the targeted area of linguistic development – the phonological system – be accelerated beyond the level which would be expected due to chronological development?

Any improvement which took place in the children's phonological ability over the treatment phase of the investigation can be determined by comparing the number of simplifying processes operating before and after treatment. Table 7 shows the number of processes present in each child's speech before and after therapy as measured by the MRP. This table shows that all children used fewer simplifying processes after treatment with a mean reduction from 6.7 to 2.5 occurrences. A Wilcoxon matched pairs signed rank test showed this to be a highly significant reduction ($p < 0.01$).

Although this result demonstrates beyond any doubt that phonological development had taken place over the treatment period, we cannot automatically assume that this change was due to the treatment provided. The children's phonological ability may have improved simply because they got older, the same progress being achieved without speech therapy.

Table 7 Number of simplifying processes used by each subject pre- and post- treatment

Subject	Number of processes	
	Pre-treatment	*Post-treatment*
1	6	1
2	8	3
3	6	5
4	7	1
5	5	2
6	8	0
7	4	2
8	10	5
9	8	4
10	4	1
11	6	2
12	8	4
13	6	2
Mean	6.7	2.5
Range	4–10	0–5

In order to try to determine whether the treatment was actually responsible for the changes we compared the pre- and post-phonological scores with the children's pre- and post-treatment scores on the BPVS. The BPVS provided a measure of another aspect of language, vocabulary, something which we would not expect to change as a result of the type of treatment provided in the study. The mean BPVS standard score before treatment was 103.6 (SD 8.55) and after treatment it was 104.5 (SD 7.95), a difference which is not significant. It does appear therefore that there was a significant change in phonological development, but no change in vocabulary development beyond that which could be expected due to age.

It is of course possible to argue that phonological development takes place on a different time scale to vocabulary development. Nevertheless the statistical results confirm our first two predictions and provide strong evidence that Metaphon treatment was responsible for accelerating phonological development in this group of children.

Although the children in this investigation appeared to be representative of the phonologically disordered population they were nevertheless a relatively small group. Furthermore they were all treated by the same therapist. Later in the chapter we describe how we have tested the effectiveness of Metaphon more extensively by involving several therapists and many more children in the second investigation.

Does Metaphon therapy specifically affect those processes which are targeted in therapy or is its effect more general?

The nature of change can be determined by comparing progress on the two treated processes and the control process for each child using the results of the MRP Monitoring Procedure. This procedure enables us to measure the percentage occurrence of each of the three processes before, during and after therapy.

These were plotted on to graphs where the vertical axis of each graph represented the percentage occurrence of each process and the horizontal axis the number of the monitoring trial.

Those graphs that showed similar patterns of change were grouped together and three groups emerged (see Figures 16, 17 and 18 for an example from each group).

Group 1 represents what can be termed the 'process specific group'. This group is characterised by reduction of percentage occurrence of both treated processes during the time that they were being targeted with no change in the untreated process. If Subject 3 (Figure 16) is taken as an example, we can see that all three processes are operating at 100% at trials one to three (the three pre-treatment trials). The percentage occurrence of the first treated process then starts to fall and is at 80% on the fourth monitoring trial. Percentage occurrence continued to fall,

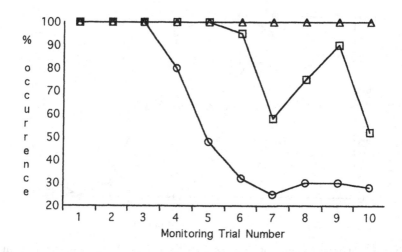

Figure 16 Typical pattern of process change. Group 1: process specific group. Subject 3. N = 5/13. ○ = Treated Process A. □ = Treated Process B. △ = Control process

and drops to about 30% on the tenth monitoring trial. Mean-while the second treated process stays constant to the sixth monitoring trial and then shows a fall rise pattern, whilst the untreated process stays at 100% occurrence throughout the pre-treatment and treatment monitoring trials. Five of the 13 children fell into this group (subjects 3, 4, 5, 7 and 8). For these children we can say that treatment had only affected those processes which were specifically targeted.

We can refer to Group 2 as the 'generalisation group'. The monitoring trial results from children in this group shows that change in process occurrence was not restricted to the treated processes but was generalised to the untreated process and all processes for this group were reduced to zero, or only minimal, occurrence. Figure 17 illustrates this pattern. There were four children in this group (subjects 1, 2, 6 and 9).

Group 3 comprises the remaining four subjects (10, 11, 12 and 13), who can be referred to as the indeterminate group. The results from these children do not fall clearly into either of the other two groups. Some reduction took place in the percentage occurrence of both treated and untreated processes for all the subjects in this group and they therefore resemble Group 2 children most closely. However, they differed from the children in Group 2 in the extent to which process occurrence decreased. Figure 18 shows a typical pattern from this group.

A feature of Group 3 is the variability of process occurrence; in

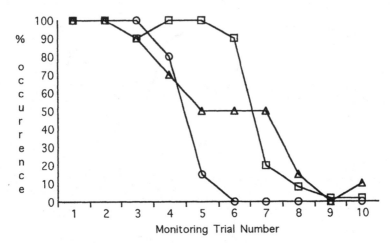

Figure 17 Typical pattern of process change. Group 2: generalisation group. Subject 1. N = 4/13. ○ = Treated Process A. □ = Treated Process B. △ = Control process

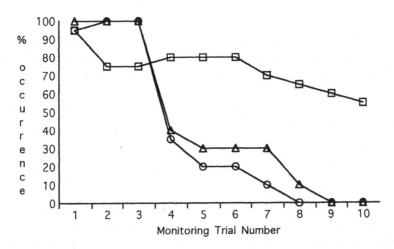

Figure 18 Typical pattern of process change. Group 3: indeterminate group. Subject 10. N = 4/13.○ = Treated Process A. □ = Treated Process B. △ = Control process

many instances a process will fall then rise and fall again. This is an indication that generalisation of the adult target is not finally determined. It is possible that the child may still be in the process of experimenting and hypothesis testing; in other words learning may still be taking place. Such a possibility accords well with theories of phonological acquisition and the pattern of learning that we would wish to emulate in treatment (see Chapter 6).

The results of the monitoring trials show that children react in different ways to Metaphon therapy. We cannot therefore provide a clearcut answer to our second question as to whether the effect of Metaphon treatment is general or specific. There are several possible reasons which might account for the variety of response patterns that emerged. We can divide these into three general categories: first, explanations that relate to the particular combinations of simplifying phonological processes the children use; second, linguistic development explanations, and third, other individual characteristics. We will consider each in turn.

The pattern of phonological change may be associated with possible interrelationships between processes. Common sense tells us that some processes are more closely related than others. Therefore treatment of one might lead to spontaneous resolution of another without treatment. For example, in the MRP we consider stopping of fricatives and stopping of affricates as two separate processes because we sometimes see children who present only with the latter. If children present in the clinic with both these processes the therapist might work first on eliminating stopping of fricatives but find that the effect of that treatment frequently results spontaneously in the resolution of stopping of affricates.

There is currently little published information about potential connections between processes beyond the very obvious ones such as the example given above. We examined the processes chosen for treatment and control for each child in this study to see if there were any similarities within, or differences between, the three groups which could provide indications of possible generalisation effects between treated and control processes. The range and combinations of processes that were chosen to act as treatment and control processes were found to be very similar for all three groups of children (Table 8).

If we look at the processes which were treated and those which acted as the control processes within each group, we can see that there are no obvious differences between the groups with one exception; there is a tendency for combinations of processes involving fricatives and affricates to be selected as treated and control processes in the generalisation and indeterminate groups (subjects 2, 9 and 12), a pattern that did not occur in the process specific group.

It does not seem possible therefore on the basis of this analysis, to explain the children's varying responses to treatment by reference to change in specific combinations of processes.

However, if we move outside the experimental situation, there does appear to be some support for the view that Metaphon has a general rather than a specific effect. For instance, when we looked at the data of the children described in Chapter 3, we found that spontaneous resolution of most processes tended to occur after specific treatment of

Table 8 Treatment and control processes used by subjects in each group

Subject	Treated Process A	Treated Process B	Control process
Group 1: Process specific			
3	Final consonant. deletion	Stopping affricates	Cluster reduction (plosive + approximant)
4	Velar fronting	Syllable initial voicing	Gliding liquids
5	Stopping fricatives	Gliding liquids	Syllable initial voicing
7	Velar fronting	Gliding liquids	Fronting (θ as f)
8	Velar fronting	Initial fricative deletion	Gliding liquids
Group 2: Generalisation			
1	Velar fronting	Stopping fricatives	Gliding liquids
2	Syllable initial voicing	Stopping fricatives	Stopping affricates
6	Palato-alveolar fronting	Stopping affricates	Gliding liquids
9	Velar fronting	Initial fricative deletion	Stopping affricates
Group 3: Indeterminate			
10	Backing (f,v → s,z)	Gliding liquids	Cluster reduction (s + plosive)
11	Stopping fricatives	Syllable initial voicing	Gliding liquids
12	Stopping fricatives	Gliding liquids	Stopping affricates
13	Syllable initial voicing	Front/back confusion	Gliding liquids

two or three had been provided. This pattern of change during treatment was typical of most children in the investigation. Changes took place over a longer time span and over more processes than the three we were concerned with during the specific treatment monitoring period of the experiment. This may well be an indication that a general increase in knowledge about the phonological aspects of language is the influencing feature of therapy rather than the specific focus on a particular process.

In the current investigation the choice of treatment and control processes was largely a clinical decision. That is, processes were chosen for treatment in relation to the perceived needs of each individual child, using the type of criteria that we referred to in Chapter 3. We feel that the generalisation effect between processes requires further investigation not only because it will increase our knowledge of how Metaphon works but also for practical and economic reasons. When the second investigation is completed we will be able to look more extensively at whether Metaphon has a general or specific effect on process change. We will also have much more information about the specific relationship between processes. It may, however, be necessary to do even further investigation which would require us to make specific predictions about generalisation effects and select processes for treatment to test these predictions.

We have been concerned above with the particular characteristics of simplifying processes. We know that there is also a developmental dimension to such processes, in that certain processes are eliminated earlier than others in the process of normal development. This developmental dimension might have had an influence on the different patterns of change that occurred.

One of the difficulties of assessing this potential influence during the period of therapy is that we lack information about children's developmental progression before they are referred to the speech therapist. We do not know, for example, whether they have already resolved some simplifying processes without treatment or whether their development is static. Monitoring trials that were administered over the pre-test period of this investigation showed that all measured processes for all children were invariably static over this period. This was a relatively short period of three or four weeks, however, and it may well be that for some, even if not all, children phonological change was taking place spontaneously but slowly. Because we lack detailed knowledge of the children's phonological development, we do not know at what stage in the resolution of a process we are intervening. We may, by good fortune, have chosen to focus on processes which were already starting to change. In that case the effect of therapy may be to accelerate and speed up such change. In other instances we may have chosen processes which the child was not ready to change and in that case overt improvement would not be so easy to achieve, though we may well be providing the child with information that will help change at a later date.

Finally, the individual characteristics of each child, such as personality, cognitive ability and motivation, will always exert some influence on the child's response to treatment. External influences such as environmental situation and factors such as length of time in treatment and attendance record which we referred to earlier will also affect the success of treatment.

We did not investigate in any great detail the relationship between individual characteristics and response to Metaphon therapy. There were, however, some interesting differences in the subjects' performance on the speech sound imitation task. On pre-therapy testing, the generalising group tended to be better imitators (significant at <0.05 on Mann-Whitney U test). It is possible to speculate that children in this group had problems which were primarily phonological and that therapy had led to reorganisation of the system with effects going beyond the targeted processes. In contrast subjects in the process specific group with poorer imitation skills may have been experiencing

some speech motor (phonetic) constraints on their speech development, possibly hindering generalisation. Further discussion on this
point can be found in Dean et al. (in press) The larger numbers of subjects in the second investigation will enable us to investigate the possible relationships between individual variation and response to therapy
in much more detail. Pursuing this line of investigation is important
because it not only provides us with general information about the success or otherwise of Metaphon therapy, but it has the potential for
increasing our knowledge of the disorder and enabling us to adapt
Metaphon to suit the specific needs of individual children, a topic that
we take up in more detail in the two final chapters.

To summarise, in response to our second question of specific versus
general change, we have to conclude that either type of change can
occur. A number of variables may be responsible for influencing how
children change. Some of these require further investigation and there
is every possibility that the results of such investigation can influence
treatment planning. Other possible factors will be less accessible to
study and will continue to have an influence on the effect of therapy
over which therapists will be able to exercise little control.

*Can concomitant changes in metalinguistic awareness provide evid-
ence about the way in which intervention influences the phonological
system?*

So far we have been able to show that phonological change took place
and we have seen that, at least to some extent, this can be attributed to
the treatment that the subjects received. We have also seen that the
nature of phonological change varied between subjects. For a substan-
tial number of the children, change was specific to the processes treated but for others it was more general. Finally, we have to consider our
third question, which is concerned with why change took place. We
have assumed that change in phonological development results from
our focus on linguistic awareness. This is a fundamental premise of
Metaphon; but we cannot presume that because change took place this
confirms our assumption that it is a result of increasing metalinguistic
awareness; hence the need for the third question.

We addressed this issue by testing children's linguistic awareness
before and after the treatment phase of the investigation. We predicted
that performance on metalinguistic tasks designed to test phonological
and communicative awareness would change more than performance
on syntactic awareness tasks.

The results of our investigation supported our predictions to a limited extent (Table 9).

Performance on the communicative awareness and phoneme segmentation tasks showed a highly significant difference pre- and post-

Table 9 Mean percentage scores for metalinguistic tasks pre- and post-treatment

Task	Percentage score		Significance
	Pre-treatment	Post-treatment	
Phoneme segment	42.4	80.2	p<0.01
Communicat. effect.	9.4	42.2	p<0.01
Sentence segment	60.1	83.9	p<0.01
Syntactic structure	62.4	68.1	not sig.

treatment, whereas performance on the syntactic awareness task was not significant. However, performance on the sentence segmentation task pre- and post-treatment also showed significant change and this did not support our predictions. However, we have to consider the nature of this task; it was intended as a measure of word awareness. It may well be that what we were assessing was an increasing awareness that speech is not a continuous stream but is composed of a series of units which can be divided into progressively smaller units. If we consider the nature of some of the activities we provide in Metaphon therapy, we should not be surprised at this result. Such an assumption would also be in accord with the theories of acquisition proposed by Peters (1983) and Waterson (1987). We also have a considerable amount of evidence that the ability to segment speech tends to show a developmental progression through word, syllable and, finally, phoneme segmentation. For example, Fox and Routh (1975) found that 3-year-olds were able to segment sentences into words but it was not until the age of five that segmentation of phonemes became an easy task for the majority of children. On the whole we can say in response to this question that change appears to be taking place in both phonological awareness and phonological ability.

Stronger evidence of a relationship between linguistic awareness and phonological change could be provided if it were possible to demonstrate an association between metalinguistic task results and phonological change after treatment. We therefore carried out statistical analysis to see if any correlation existed. The result was a low positive but non-significant correlation between the two measures. This lack of significant correlation might arise because we are not measuring like with like. The processes investigated in this study were different for each child but in most cases they were operating at 100% occurrence and therefore shared a common baseline from which to measure change. However, each child had different scores on the metalinguistic tasks; that is they had different levels of linguistic awareness, as measured by these tasks, at the start of the investigation. It was not therefore possible to establish a common baseline for these tasks from which change could be measured. Had it been possible to devise met-alinguistic tasks where the children all started from the same level of ability a significant correlation between phonological development and metalinguistic ability may have resulted. The different levels of ability on metalinguistic tasks are to be expected. We discussed in Chapter 4 that even though the phonologically disordered population as a group has inferior metalinguistic ability to normally developing children, there are considerable variations within each group. Because of these variations we have to conclude that poor linguistic awareness is neither a necessary nor sufficient explanation of delayed phonological development.

We have continued to look at the relationship between linguistic awareness and the results of Metaphon therapy in our second investigation. The greater numbers of subjects involved in this study will enable us to carry out more extensive statistical analysis to examine possible relationships in this area. We have also designed this study to enable us to examine the relative contribution to phonological change of the different aspects of metalinguistic awareness that we focus on at different stages of Metaphon.

During this discussion of the first efficacy study we have referred to the issues that require further investigation. We will finish this chapter by describing how we designed the second investigation to address these issues.

The Second Efficacy Study

Three main questions are being addressed in this investigation:

1. Can the effectiveness of Metaphon be demonstrated in a larger group of therapists and children?
2. Are both phases of Metaphon required to bring about phonological change?
3. What factors contribute to variations in response to therapy?

We will take each question in turn.

Can the Effectiveness of Metaphon be Demonstrated in a Larger Group of Therapists and Children?

Although the results of the first investigation supported our clinical impressions that Metaphon therapy was an effective therapeutic procedure for phonologically disordered children we did not feel that a sample of 13 children treated by a single therapist gave us sufficiently robust evidence to recommend this therapy procedure unequivocally. More information from a larger group of subjects was required.

We recruited twenty qualified speech and language therapists from six different regions of the United Kingdom to participate in the second study. These therapists differ widely in their training and experience: some are experienced Metaphon users whilst others were new to the approach at the start of the investigation. Regardless of their existing experience we gave all of them three days training at the start of the project to enable them to learn how to use Metaphon therapy and to familiarise them with the assessments used in the investigation. We maintain contact with the therapists throughout the investigation and frequently video their therapy sessions to monitor their interpretation and presentation of Metaphon.

We hope that about 50 children will have participated in the study by the time it is completed. The final number will depend on the number of suitable subjects referred to each therapist. We are using the same criteria as in the first study to select suitable subjects, with one addition; in order to provide a standardised measure of sound system development we are also testing the children on the Edinburgh Articulation Test (EAT) (Anthony et al., 1971). To qualify for inclusion in the investigation the children require a Standard Score of 85 or less (1 standard deviation) on this test.

Are Both Phases of Metaphon Required to Bring About Phonological Change?

The design of the first study did not lend itself to determining whether children need to progress through all phases of Metaphon therapy to achieve phonological change. It is possible that they may only need information about the sound system of their native language, Phase 1 of Metaphon, to start the process of phonological change or they may also need information about their communicative competence, provided by Phase 2 of Metaphon. This is an important question to ask both from the point of view of understanding how Metaphon works and also in terms of the question of therapeutic efficiency. The number of therapy sessions required may be reduced if we can demonstrate that children do not need all phases of Metaphon. This is an issue that has been raised by therapists other than ourselves who are using Metaphon in their clinical practice (see, for example, Howard and Hesketh, 1993).

So that we could find out whether children require both phases of Metaphon the experiment has been designed so that each therapist selects four or eight children for the investigation. The children are randomly assigned to the following four groups (one or two children per group):

Group 1: Treatment condition: 6 sessions (3 hours) of Phase 1 of Metaphon
Group 2: Treatment condition: 10 sessions (5 hours) of Phase 1 and

Phase 2 of Metaphon
Group 3: No treatment condition, untreated control group for Group 1
Group 4: No treatment condition, untreated control group for Group 2.

Including untreated control groups in the investigation also allows us to control for the effect of maturation by comparing treated and untreated groups of children, something that was not possible in the first investigation.

A series of assessments are administered to all subjects before the start of the therapy period. Readministration of some of the assessments then takes place at the end of therapy for the treated children and after a corresponding time interval for the control groups, that is, there is a six or ten week interval between pre- and post-testing for Groups 3 and 4 respectively. We should stress that no child is denied therapy. Children in the control groups are given therapy as soon as the assessments have been readministered.

The therapists select one process for treatment and one to act as an untreated control for each Group 1 and Group 2 child, and two control processes for each Group 3 and Group 4 child. The screening and probes sections of the MRP (Dean et al., 1990) are used to select these processes and measure phonological change.

Treatment sessions follow the same pattern as those in the first study, that is, they take place once a week and last for approximately 30 minutes.

A comparison of the very early results from this investigation show that some children in both treated groups are demonstrating marked phonological change. There is a tendency for Group 2 children to show more generalised change than Group 1 children. This of course may be a reflection of the length of time elapsing between pre- and post-treatment assessment. At this very early stage in the analysis of the results the most we can say is that at least for some children providing them with information about the sound system of their native language appears to be sufficient to accelerate phonological change.

What Factors Contribute to Variations in Response to Therapy?

We spent some time earlier in this chapter examining possible reasons for the different response patterns we observed in the children in the first study. This larger investigation provides us with the opportunity to specifically investigate some of the factors we discussed earlier.

Information about factors that might contribute to a child's response to therapy is obtained by looking at the relationship between individual characteristics and response to therapy. We are assessing a large number of such characteristics in this investigation, including measures of speech processing ability, linguistic awareness and aspects of cognition. We will look at each of these three groups in turn.

Metalinguistic Ability

We are using the three metalinguistic tasks specifically designed for the investigation which we referred to in Chapter 3. The tasks assess awareness of rhyme, awareness of word initial phonemes and word order in sentences. Care was taken to see that all the tasks used simple instructions, involved activities which were interesting to the children and were quick and easy to administer by the therapists.

Speech Processing

We saw earlier that there appeared to be a tendency for imitation ability to be associated with differences in response to Metaphon in the first efficacy study. We have included an imitation task in the assessment battery of this investigation, and extended the assessment of motor speech ability further with a polysyllabic repetition task. Both assessments were devised for the investigation.

We have also devised an auditory discrimination task for the investigation which assesses the children's discriminatory ability in relation to the type of errors which occur in their own speech.

Cognition

The British Picture Vocabulary Scales (Dunn et al., 1982) are being used to measure verbal intelligence to enable us to examine whether there is any relationship between this variable and response to therapy.

We are also using two measures of cognitive style in the assessment battery for this investigation; the Kansas Reflection Impulsivity Pre School Scales (KRISP) (Wright, Gaughan and McClanachan, 1978) and a motor inhibition task (Draw a line) (Maccoby et al., 1965). These assessments have been included to enable us to find out whether reflective children do better than impulsive children with Metaphon therapy. We did not specifically assess cognitive style in the first study but it was noticeable that the therapist who treated the children made frequent reference to their behaviour on this dimension in relation to how they responded to therapy. It might be expected that, because Metaphon encourages children to reflect about language, differences in outcome might reflect children's behaviour on these reflection impulsivity measures. Information about the relationship between response to therapy and cognitive style is potentially of considerable practical value. If it is found that reflective children respond more quickly to

Metaphon than impulsive children, there is further potential for adapting Metaphon to meet specific child needs. We will not be in a position to provide any answer to this our third question, the effect of individual characteristics on response to therapy, until our research is complete and we have carried out statistical analysis on the results.

We hope that when the analysis of the results of this current investigation are published they will offer increased opportunities to make Metaphon as effective and efficient as possible by tailoring it to match what is known about each individual child.

In the next chapter we look at the ways in which Metaphon therapy might be adapted in different ways for children with disordered phonology, and provide some information about how Metaphon has been used with other client groups, and in languages other than English.

Chapter 9
Wider Applications of Metaphon

In this chapter we examine the possibilities of modifying the customary Metaphon approach to suit the specific needs of sub-groups of children with disordered phonology. We then go on to discuss the use of Metaphon therapy beyond the clinical setting and the client group for which it was originally designed.

In our descriptions of theory applied to practice we confined ourselves to one specific group, the pre-school phonologically disordered child, in one pattern of therapeutic organisation – individual, once weekly, treatment. Metaphon was originally conceived to meet the particular needs of this group within the constraints of an existing setting and it is for this group in this setting that we have applied Metaphon most extensively. We have, however, frequently been asked if the Metaphon principles can be more widely applied to a range of phonologically disordered children in different clinical settings, or to other client groups.

Because Metaphon is essentially a method of working, rather than a specific treatment programme, it is appropriate to consider how Metaphon as presented so far might be extended or modified. Our discussion of the wider application of Metaphon will include suggestions for its use with phonologically disordered children in settings other than one to one individual therapy, the adaptation of Metaphon for other client groups and the use of Metaphon therapy with children speaking languages other than English. Before we discuss these topics, however, we want to spend some time looking at possible modifications to the Metaphon approach for what we will describe as potential 'sub-groups' within the phonologically disordered population. We will concentrate particularly on children who might require opportunities to develop their phonetic (speech motor) skills.

171

Therapy for Sub-groups of Children with Disordered Phonology

As we said in Chapter 2, children with a diagnosis of phonological disorder are probably a heterogeneous population with regard to the explanation of their speech difficulties. One of the basic aims of the Metaphon approach is to provide therapy which is as efficient and effective as possible. One way of fulfilling this aim is to adapt Metaphon to individual children's speech processing limitations.

The first step in this adaptation is to determine what these constraints might be. Potential limitations may be revealed by assessment procedures or by response to therapy. We saw from the results of the first efficacy study, described in the previous chapter, that there were marked differences in the children's response to therapy and such differences may at least in part be attributed to the children's differential underlying competencies in speech processing. We can use information from the study to illustrate this possibility by comparing performance on the speech sound imitation task with therapy outcome. On pre-therapy testing the generalisation outcome group tended to be better imitators ($p<0.05$, on Mann–Whitney U test) than the other children. Dean et al. (in press) suggest that this difference is consistent with the view that the problems of the children in this outcome group were primarily phonological and that therapy resulted in effective reorganisation of the system beyond the specifically targeted processes. In contrast, the subjects in the process specific outcome group, who were poorer imitators, may have been experiencing some speech motor (phonetic level) constraints on their speech development. (See for instance Example 1 in Chapter 3, David.)

If, as seems highly likely, certain speech processing constraints affect response to therapy it is appropriate that we should adapt therapy to meet the needs of individual children. We will look at some possible modifications later in the chapter, after we have discussed the assessment and nature of possible limitations in a little more detail.

The adaptation of Metaphon therapy will be achieved most efficiently if we are able to determine possible constraints before commencing therapy rather than basing all modifications on the child's response to therapy. Potential constraints will not be discovered without a comprehensive assessment. We stressed the need for the assessment of all levels of speech processing and commended the assessment approach of Stackhouse and Wells (1993) in Chapter 2. Unfortunately, although there are promising developments in this area, some of the assessments currently available to the practising clinician may not provide the depth of information that is required and they are of limited use in determining the most appropriate intervention procedures. There is, however, some experimental work which looks at the speech process-ing abilities of children with speech and language difficulties. Such investigations provide us with the opportunity to suggest testable hypo-thetical modifications to Metaphon therapy.

Speech Motor Control Constraints

The status of the speech motor control of children with disordered phonology has received more attention than other aspects of speech processing. The evidence from these investigations suggests:

> ... the possibility that at least some children with speech and language disor-ders may have poorer speech motor abilities than normal children and that deficits in the fine motor co-ordination skills which underlie speech produc-tion may be implicated in children's speech disorders. (Dean et al., in press.)

Some of the most recent investigation in this area has been carried out by Waters (1992), who investigated the possibility that slow matura-tion of speech motor control may underlie phonological delay. She compared the speech timing characteristics of groups of normal pre-school children, age matched phonologically delayed children and nor-mal adult speakers, by carrying out spectrographic measurement of phrase and segment duration and temporal variations in repetitions of an experimental phrase. As a group the phonologically delayed chil-dren were found to have significantly slower speech rates than the nor-mally developing children. There was also a trend towards longer phrase and segment duration in the data from the delayed children. Since speed and consistency are regarded as indices of maturity in the development of speech motor performance these results lend support to the view that speech motor co-ordination and control may be less mature in some phonologically disordered children than in their peers.

The implications of these results for Metaphon therapy are consid-ered by Waters (1992) and Dean et al. (in press). Although sound pro-duction is never the direct focus of therapy in Metaphon, these authors believe that this approach can be an effective medium to enable those children who require opportunities to develop their speech motor skills to do so. Phase 1 of Metaphon provides the opportunity for the child to play, and experiment, with speech sound production. Encouragement is given to produce a variety of non-speech and speech sounds which fall into certain categories depending upon the simplify-ing process which is being targeted. Dean et al. suggest:

> ... that during these activities the child is gradually discovering, strengthen-ing and automising the processing of motor plans which match particular perceptual categories of speech sounds. This gradual motor learning must depend on repeated opportunities to experience the combined auditory,

proprioceptive and kinaesthetic feedback associated with particular vocal tract configurations, reinforced by external feedback from the therapist.

Phase 2 of Metaphon therapy provides the opportunity to enable the child to move towards adult realisation of the target contrast in a communicative situation. In terms of Hewlett's model (described in Chapter 2) such a learning situation, which focuses on communicative awareness, will raise awareness of mismatch between the child's own and the adult target and encourage revision towards new, more appropriate motor plans. An essential aspect in bringing about these changes is the nature of the graded feedback provided by the therapist which encourages the child to make further attempts to achieve the adult target forms. The aim is that through repeated use in activities during Phase 2 Sentence Level these revisions gradually become more automatic.

Some support for the view that Metaphon is helpful in overcoming phonetic limitations can be derived from a comparison of the pre and post intervention scores on the consonant imitation task in the first efficacy study. There was a highly significant difference in these scores ($p < 0.01$, Wilcoxon Signed Rank test). This result suggests that imitation ability, and by implication motor speech processing, was facilitated by Metaphon therapy despite the fact that direct speech sound imitation plays no part in this kind of therapy.

Some practical adaptations to the customary Metaphon activities are suggested by this speculative explanation of how Metaphon therapy might be operating to bring about change for those children whose phonological difficulties have their origins in motor processing constraints. There is a need, first of all, to encourage and allow ample opportunity for motor exploration and practice. The nature of the child's limitations suggests that therapy will have to be planned in the expectation that it will be necessary to focus explicitly on each target contrast in turn. We should probably not expect generalisation of learning to lead to elimination of other simplifying processes for this group of children. Care will have to be taken to ensure that activities and materials focus on and encourage exploration of all phonemes affected by the targeted process.

Dean, Anderson and Waters (1992) suggest that in some cases in addition to adaptation Metaphon might need to be extended for children with motor processing constraints to give specific information about the articulatory specifications of sounds. They suggest a more extensive and explicit vocabulary for describing the properties of sounds and the possibility of using visual referent cards to illustrate individual sounds within the target class. Similar suggestions are made later in this chapter in relation to the adaptation of Metaphon for use with cleft palate children.

Suggestions for the adaptation of Metaphon for other potential sub-groups of specifically phonologically disordered children can only be speculative in the absence, to date, of experimental evidence of how these groups might be constituted. On the basis of the potential levels of breakdown in speech processing that we referred to in Chapter 2 it is possible that there are sub-groups of children with auditory discrimination difficulties, of various kinds, and others that have poor phonological awareness.

Auditory Discrimination Constraints

Therapy for those children with demonstrated auditory discrimination problems might include additional opportunities for taking the role of the listener in Phase 1 and using activities that provided optimum opportunity to recognise, match and categorise sounds in graded activities which ensure step by step progress from Phoneme to Word Level during Phase 1. It is essential to stress that for these children a detailed assessment of specific discrimination difficulties is required so that therapy can be precisely targeted.

Metaphon in its customary form, as described in Chapter 7, might appear to be ideally suited to children who are found to have specific metaphonological limitations, but even for these children it should be possible to enhance learning in this particular direction. These children may need more general metalinguistic activities which might precede or go alongside the information they are given about the specific sound contrasts which forms the main focus of their therapy. Increased exposure to nursery and nonsense rhymes, simple rhyming and segmentation activities of the kind we suggest later in this chapter may enhance their metalinguistic awareness and facilitate the effectiveness of the specific activities being used to bring about phonological change.

So far we have made some general suggestions for adapting Metaphon to potential speech processing weaknesses. It is inevitable that response to therapy will also be influenced by other individual child characteristics. We have already stressed the importance of planning Metaphon therapy to suit each child's individual needs in terms of their personality, interests and motivation and we have suggested a variety of activities that can be adapted to these differences. In our current efficacy study we are carrying out investigations of learning style as part of our assessment battery. We hope that these tests will show us whether children tend to be reflective or impulsive in their approach to tasks and we can then compare this measure with their respective responses to Metaphon therapy. As Metaphon is directed towards encouraging children to reflect about aspects of language it might be expected that children who are shown to be generally reflective might respond rather better to this type of therapy than children who have a tendency to be impulsive. If our results support this supposition it may be advisable to build into Metaphon activities which encourage the child to be more reflective, and therefore less impulsive, before starting to encourage specific reflection on language.

Group Therapy and Metaphon

So far we have considered Metaphon therapy only in a one to one situation of child and therapist. Metaphon is being used increasingly in group work with phonologically disordered children with some promising results. The following account of using Metaphon with groups of children is based on information supplied by Carolyn Anderson, and Julie Williams and her colleagues.

There are two main reasons given for preferring to work with children in groups rather than individually. First, it is argued that it is an economical way of providing therapy. For example, if the same results can be achieved by treating five children in a group for eight one hour sessions compared to treating the same five children individually in eight half hour sessions (the average length of treatment time spent treating one process in the first efficacy study) the total treatment time is more than halved. Second, groups lend themselves to the 'block' pattern of therapy and there is an increasing trend towards this type of provision. In 'block' provision therapists treat in one clinical setting, such as a specific school, before moving on to the next setting for which they provide a service. In addition therapists who work in paediatric speech and language therapy services that have taken an administrative decision to treat their clients in groups and provide little or no individual therapy will have no option other than to use Metaphon in a group setting.

Opinions vary about the age at which children should be included in Metaphon groups. Some therapists run groups just for pre-school children, whilst others run groups for school-aged children as well. It is suggested that group work might be most successful if restricted to children from 4 years of age upwards because they will normally have experience of a nursery setting by this age and will therefore be accustomed to working in groups. However, some pre-school groups contain children aged from 3;6. Age will not be the only criterion for selection, however, and this may also depend on other factors such as the level of social and emotional development, the severity of the disorder and concomitant problems.

The size of the group is to some extent dependent on the number of adults – therapists, helpers, or parents – who are available. As a general guideline five or six children per group with a ratio of one adult to two or three children seems to be an ideal size to provide sufficient individual attention and keep the children actively involved in therapy activities. Group sessions tend to follow the once weekly pattern suggested for individual Metaphon treatment but usually last for a minimum of one hour rather than thirty minutes.

When planning the composition and purpose of a group it seems customary in most cases to run groups for specific processes, that is a fronting/backing group, a stopping group and so on. But some services run what are described as 'general phonology groups' and children usually attend one of these before they are enrolled in a process specific group. These general groups provide only Phase 1 therapy and focus on different processes, targeting each process separately for two weeks at a time. For example, two weeks targeting stopping, two targeting fronting/backing and two targeting voicing contrasts.

Planning a series of group sessions to target a specific process will probably follow the progression of Metaphon used in the individual therapy outline that we described in Chapter 7. However, as group sessions are longer, short breaks at intervals between therapy activities may be needed. The children will also need to get to know one another, to facilitate group participation, so some time must be allowed for familiarisation activities. The basic aims at each level will remain the same as those for individual work.

In individual treatment, progression through Metaphon is continually being revised and tailored to suit the child's responses. Such constant adaptation is, of course, not possible during group work. However, it is essential that we respond to each child's needs to ensure maximum therapeutic effectiveness. Careful monitoring of reaction to therapy is essential, for example when deciding to move from level to level or from Phase 1 to Phase 2. It is suggested that the therapy plan should allow for the opportunity to work with each child individually for a short period at this time, so that discussion and therapy activities can be conducted according to individual needs. The main requirement for this crucial stage of therapy is to proceed at the individual's own pace and this be difficult to accommodate within the context of a group.

There are several different ways of coping with individual differences in response to therapy within a group setting. These may include taking the whole group back a stage, splitting the group for specific activities, providing some children with a combination of individual therapy and group activities, or abandoning group work altogether for an individual child.

Decisions about which, if any, of these strategies are undertaken will of course depend on the nature of the responses to therapy and resources available. Taking the whole group back a little is a suitable strategy if progression through the stages is going a little too quickly for more than one child. It is an easy matter to introduce an extra lower level activity, such as an extra Concept Level activity in the later stages of therapy. The role of therapist feedback is as crucial in group therapy as it is in individual therapy. Careful control of the speaker/listener role of each child, and extra attention to the nature of feedback to the child who appears to be simply rather slower than the rest, presents no difficulty.

Splitting the group will be a suitable strategy if some of the children within the group appear to have difficulty in producing specific speech sounds at Phoneme Level. This type of difficulty may be an indication of the motor processing, phonetic level problems we referred to above and may further reflect the fact that phonological disorder can be influenced by a variety of other constraints. Such children may require 'branch' programmes at the same level as other Metaphon activities. These activities can be given to a sub-group who will then return to the main group for other activities.

Splitting the group at Phase 1 Word Level and using different sets of minimal pairs to accommodate children who are exhibiting the simplifying process in different word positions might also be a strategy that can be employed in the search for more efficient therapy. The sub-groups can then be successfully re-integrated into the whole group where games such as lotto and other minimal pair activities, carefully designed and manipulated, can be used to cover the needs of all the children.

Most of the activities used with individual children in Metaphon therapy can be adapted for groups and there are many games which are more suited to group work. These activities are often very simple, requiring little equipment and keeping the focus of the task direct and explicit. An adaptation of the 'statues' game provides one example. It involves the group walking around the room in a circle until the leader says 'Stop'. At this point everyone stands as still as possible and the one that moves first is chosen to do the task. The task chosen will depend on the stage the group has reached in therapy. For example, at Phase 1 Concept Level it will be carrying out an appropriate activity and at Phase 1 Word Level categorising the sound in a minimal pair word. Once the task is completed the child then chooses how the group will go around the circle, hopping, skipping etc., and the game is continued.

Other activities for specific processes which are particularly suitable for group work include the following suggestions. Groups working on the long/short contrast might dress up in long/short clothes, or feed a dog (one of the adults or children might like to be the dog) long and short bones. For the back/front contrast chairs can be made into trains or buses, the children can be passengers who sit on front or back seats. Bands with noisy/whisper instruments provide a good group activity for children working on the voicing contrast.

Phase 2 Sentence Level activities for all processes can be made very interesting if the instructions are personalised. For example, the first instruction might be – 'John pick up toe/dough', John carries out the activity then passes on the message – 'Mary pick up toe/dough', and so on. These are just a few suggested adaptations to activities for group work. We are sure that therapists will be able to adapt many of the activities we suggested in Chapter 7 for use in a group setting.

We referred earlier to adult helpers in the groups. If possible, time should be set apart before and during the group programme for explanation and discussion with the helpers about the therapy method that is being used, particularly if parents are involved. Learning about the method will also take place through experience. Typically, if parents accompany their children to the group, each child works beside his or her parent, and all adults and children are included in the activities. Phase 1 activities up to Word Level may be self explanatory to the adults in the group, but many of them will require information about what sounds fall into what categories and what features are responsible for sound changes. The therapist should make the aims of therapy explicit to parents before each session and/or follow up with a hand out after the session. Working with parents in this way has many advantages not least because they are able to observe the constructive feedback the therapist uses. The therapist can also encourage the parents to use the same type of feedback at home between sessions. At Phase 2 Word Level 'secret messages' require some preparatory explanation, demonstration and practice in order to ensure that each parent knows how to incorporate the appropriate feedback into the game.

In order to maximise the learning environment in group work some therapists give helpers specific information about the way in which they might encourage responses from the individual children they have responsibility for. For instance, if the aim of the activity is to identify and label a sound as long/short or front/back, the leader explains the activity to the group and then produces a sound for each child to identify. Helpers are asked to use the time when the group leader is talking to another child to speak quietly to their own child and ask 'What do you think?' In this way the child is encouraged to be actively involved throughout the activity.

We have heard of several therapists who run Metaphon groups following the format we have described. But we know of no published assessment and evaluation of the results of group therapy with the exception of Dean, Anderson and Waters (1992) who report significant change ($p < 0.05$) in phonological output in a group of children who participated in a group treatment programme. Some preliminary information from Williams (personal communication) is also encouraging. She reports considerable success with four out of six children in a general phonology group lasting five weeks. In a stopping group for school aged children, again lasting five weeks, the same therapist reports that three out of five children achieved consistent adult targets at Phase 2

Sentence Level. We look forward to more detailed information about the outcomes of Metaphon groups. Meanwhile, we have received favourable clinical impressions about the value of Metaphon groups. Therapists using group settings feel that it is often a preferable alternative to individual treatment as it has been shown to provide an effective learning environment for selected clients and an efficient use of therapists' clinical time. The group environment can provide additional opportunities to enhance awareness as it allows children to reflect on other children's communication attempts as well as their own. There have also been suggestions that the group environment usually promotes active involvement and motivation to learn. The influence of peers in encouraging imitation and competition should not be underestimated here.

Using Metaphon for group treatment has, as we have seen, enthusiastic adherents and there are several potential advantages to adopting such an approach. Economical considerations are perhaps uppermost, but in some instances group work may have additional learning advantages over individual therapy. There is no doubt that the Metaphon approach can lend itself well to group work and we would like to encourage further development in this area. It is, however, important to measure the success of Metaphon group therapy in the same way that the use of this approach in one to one settings has been evaluated. A start has been made on this but more work is required; when more results are available we will be able to compare quantity and quality of phonological change in both settings. Therapists will then be in a position to assess the relevant advantages of both possibilities. Preferably the decision as to which approach to choose will be based on the specific needs of each individual child but particular policies and economic considerations may overshadow such decision making. If this is the case, as we have seen, Metaphon can be adapted to meet such constraints.

Using Metaphon with Younger and Older Children

There will be some instances when the conventional method of providing Metaphon therapy either in an individual or group setting will not be appropriate. Some children, particularly those with specific developmental language disorders below the age of 3;6, may be unable to respond to the structured therapy situation, or it may not be possible to provide such a regime. In these situations we would suggest that therapists could explore the possibility of a more general, less formal approach to developing phonological awareness.

Many simple rhyming activities can be used with younger children such as participation in rhyming action games, rhyming snap and the 'Ed game'. In this game the children are asked to decide what words sound the same as the puppet's name 'Ed' (see Read, 1978). The game can of course be repeated using any name that provides a range of rhyme matching opportunities. There are many simple games of this kind, some of them within the capabilities of two year olds. Therapists can provide a collection of suggestions for parents and nursery school teachers. We know that children find these activities very enjoyable and we have evidence that using such activities can lead to encouraging phonological development without direct speech therapy intervention.

We have touched upon appropriate strategies for older children with disordered phonology earlier in the book. Here we should simply like to reiterate that phonological knowledge can be increased by the use of orthographic representations. The use of separate letters is particularly useful for helping children to see how both spoken and written words are composed of smaller elements. Orthographic representations help children to realise that manipulation of these smaller elements results in changes in sound and meaning. Use of visual symbols can be combined with more specific discussion of the nature of language and the use of more sophisticated metalinguistic games. Many of the activities that are recommended for children with reading and writing difficulties may also be useful for increasing phonological awareness in older speech disordered children. Snowling (1985) offers various suggestions. Liaison with the children's teachers is of course important when a speech therapist is working with school age children. It is desirable that the same terms are used for letters and sounds to avoid potential confusion. Discussion between teacher and therapist will facilitate the choice of the most appropriate labels.

We believe that encouraging phonological awareness need not be confined to the speech clinic and the speech and language therapist. We suggest that the specific Metaphon activities we have described in this book can also be used by parents and other carers with suitable guidance about their purpose. The parents of the children we see in our clinic are always encouraged to carry out these activities between weekly clinic visits. We believe that it should be possible to extend the principle of parents as therapists using the Metaphon approach, allowing for greater intervals between clinic visits. Such a regime, however, would require very careful planning and a willingness on the part of the clinician to allocate time to discussing with parents the nature of the problem and the principles and aims of Metaphon.

We can see therefore that it is worth exploring other ways of developing phonological knowledge and that Metaphon activities can be used in ways that are different to those we have described in detail earlier in this book. We would, however, wish to caution that such tasks should not be divorced from considering the learning theory that is such an important aspect of Metaphon. We have stressed throughout that we believe the learning and adoption of adult phonological rules by the phonologically disordered child is a gradual process. Metaphon was designed specifically to facilitate learning – it does not teach pronunciation skills. The children need time to explore, experiment with and assimilate new information if they are to achieve adult phonological rules. We believe, and our experimental results and clinical experience recommend, that Metaphon is likely to be most effective in a once weekly or at most twice weekly treatment regime. As a consequence it is economically as well as therapeutically attractive to the busy clinician. However, there may be a place for Metaphon as part of an intensive programme, where it can be used alongside other activities.

Application to Other Client Groups

So far we have looked at Metaphon for children whose difficulties appear either to be confined to the phonological level of language or to be part of a more general developmental language delay. We would now like to turn to the possible application of Metaphon principles to other client groups. These applications may be better appreciated if we repeat the basic Metaphon principles. Metaphon is concerned with:

1. Increasing knowledge of language and communication;
2. Providing a learning environment which facilitates the increase of this knowledge;
3. Utilising this knowledge to enhance communicative ability.

We would argue that these principles can be applied to any individual who has an ability to learn and who wishes to be a more effective communicator. We have reports so far of these principles being applied with clients with acquired language disorders, congenital and acquired hearing loss, adults with learning disabilities and cleft palate children. Of course the sort of knowledge to be acquired, the nature of the learning environment and methods of utilising linguistic knowledge will vary according to each client's specific needs and abilities.

We can illustrate this wider application by looking at children with congenital hearing loss and cleft palate.

Metaphon with Hearing Impaired Children

Children with congenital hearing loss will need information not only about the segmental phonological level of language but also about non-segmental features such as intonation and volume. Knowledge of phonemes has to be provided by replacing or supplementing the auditory channel with information through other sensory channels. Phase 1 activities of Metaphon are extended by focusing very specifically on the contrasts between phonetic features of frication and stopping and the use of labels which focus more directly on features such as 'nose sounds' and 'no nose sounds'. It has been found that children frequently comment or ask questions using these terms and in this way reinforce their own learning, for example 'has /z/ got voice?' Phase 2 has been found to be particularly valuable in revealing to hearing impaired children why hearing people misunderstand them and why speech intelligibility is important. Once knowledge of this kind has been acquired, hearing impaired children are in a better position to communicate more effectively, by monitoring their pronunciation and developing repair strategies using their enhanced sensitivity to the responses of their listeners.

In addition to the different knowledge that has to be acquired and employed, there is another difference between using Metaphon for specifically phonologically disordered children and for children with congenital hearing impairment. Phonologically disordered children are likely to transcend their communication difficulties in a relatively short time. For children with congenital hearing impairment, and some other client groups, active monitoring of their speech and language output will be a permanent feature of their communication strategies. But we believe that Metaphon, by making the monitoring process explicit and by providing specific tools for maximising communicative competence, can help to make communication more effective.

Using Metaphon with Cleft Palate Children

Metaphon has been successfully adapted for use, in conjunction with articulation therapy, for children with cleft palate. Kim Harland has been at the forefront of this adaptation and the information which follows has been supplied by her.

Metaphon has been used with two distinct groups within this population: children with phoneme specific velopharyngeal incompetence and a group of cleft palate children presenting with other sound system problems. We will describe the work with children with phoneme specific velopharyngeal incompetence in some detail (further information about this group can be found in Harland and Albery (in preparation)). We will then look briefly at cleft palate children with other sound system problems.

Children with phoneme specific velopharyngeal incompetence are those cleft children who replace one or more pairs of fricatives/affricates with nasal fricatives. Velopharyngeal function for all other sounds is normal. The age of the children treated using Metaphon in this group ranges from 3 years upwards. The role of Metaphon for this group is seen as an adjunct to traditional articulation therapy based on the principles of motor learning.

It is appropriate to return to Hewlett's model (Chapter 2) to consider where the level of breakdown in word production is occurring for these children and how this influences the type of therapy that is required. These children's difficulties originate at the 'vocal tract shape/movement level' of the model. Therapy therefore, in addition to fulfilling the three conditions required for therapy for specifically phonologically disordered children listed on page 60, must also fulfil Hewlett's fourth condition – the implementation of targets at speed and in a variety of phonetic contexts. Articulation therapy therefore remains essential for eliciting sounds with cleft palate children. Such therapy enables the child to search for the correct target and rehearse that target in nonsense environments; this provides a variety of phonetic contexts, giving the child the opportunity to fix and stabilise the target.

The Metaphon approach may be used alongside instrumental feedback, such as electropalatography and computer software, for cleft palate children. The 'Micronose' computer software package has been found to be particularly useful for children with phoneme specific velopharyngeal incompetence. 'Micronose' software gives the child visual information in relation to nose and mouth sounds by using a hand held acoustic module which is placed on the child's upper lip. Cartoon drawings are displayed on the computer alongside the signal from the acoustic module to provide encouragement and visual feedback of nasal tone to the child.

The concepts and labels that are used with cleft palate children, like those used with hearing impaired children, tend to directly reflect the contrast that is being targeted. The contrast between nasal and oral sounds is most frequently referred to as 'nose versus mouth', and the labels 'Mr Nose' and 'Mr Mouth' are used in therapy activities. However, in common with the usual practice in Metaphon, the children are also encouraged to discuss the concept and decide if they would prefer another label, and if so what. Some of the labels suggested by the children treated by Harland include 'bubble' versus 'no bubble', 'snort' versus 'no snort' and 'tickle/itch' versus 'no tickle/itch'. We would argue that if children are encouraged to provide their own labels in this way the task of making contrasts in their speech becomes more salient and helps motivation. The children's descriptions and labels also have the added advantage of providing some information about what features of the sound contrast are perceived as most distinctive by an individual child. The therapist can use this information to tailor therapeutic activities and material precisely to the child's perceptions.

Metaphon therapy for cleft children follows the same pattern of progressive stages described in Chapter 7. Activities which relate to the oral nasal distinction at Concept Level tend to be related closely to facial features and may include jigsaw faces of animals, people and monsters and misfit/funny faces. At non-speech Sound Level 'Mr Nose' sounds are likely to be sneezing, snoring and grunting and 'Mr Mouth' sounds laughing, crying and coughing. Figure 19 shows illustrations that are used to represent 'Mr Nose' and 'Mr Mouth' (these pictures may also be enlarged so that the mouth and nose spaces can serve as posting boxes). At Phoneme Level the sound contrast used is nasal versus oral fricatives. Nasal stops are not introduced.

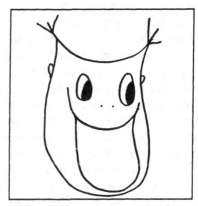

Figure 19 Referent cards for cleft palate children, 'Mr Nose/Mr Mouth'

There are two distinctive and specific differences between Metaphon for specifically phonologically disordered children and cleft palate children with phoneme specific velopharyngeal incompetence. First, at Phase 1 Word Level non-meaningful minimal pairs, that is nonsense syllables, for example [ɳ̊ˤi] versus /si/, will be used initially to develop the required skill of detecting the phonemes in words. Second, because nasal fricatives are not used in English a nasal/oral fricative pair with meaning cannot be used during Phase 2 to facilitate communicative competence. Instead, meaningful minimal pairs such as voiceless/voiced **oral** fricative pairs such as 'Sue/zoo', which are natural partner targets, are used as the 'secret messages'. If the child uses a nasal fricative ('Mr Nose' sound) the listener will not understand the message because it could be representing either the voiceless target 'Sue' or the voiced target 'zoo'. In other words the use of these voiceless/voiced oral fricative pairs as 'secret messages' demonstrates ambiguity, and communication breakdown to the child when a nasal fricative is used. Feedback from the therapist will then be along the lines of 'I'm not sure what you want as I heard a 'Mr Nose' sound'.

Another more general difference during Phase 2 when adapting Metaphon for cleft palate children is the probable need to refer to the affected aspect of production as well as communicative effectiveness. Feedback about production can be given, for example, through visual referents which will help the children to alter their articulatory attempts in order to communicate more successfully. For young children the visual referent might be a face with a mouth and a nose and stickers are added to the mouth and nose, depending on the nature of the child's production. The child can place the stickers in relation to their own production to encourage them to self monitor their performance and self correct when necessary. Older children can monitor themselves when reading, and put Mr Nose and Mr Mouth stickers on words containing fricatives depending on whether they judge their fricative production to be nasal or oral.

Other common phonological output errors of children with cleft palate, apart from phoneme specific velopharyngeal incompetence, are backing of bilabials/alveolars to velar place of articulation and glottal realisations. Metaphon can be incorporated into the treatment programme alongside articulation therapy for children from three years upwards. The role of Metaphon in treating these children follows the general pattern described for the other cleft palate group. The labels used to illustrate the concepts are usually the more familiar ones of front/back, present/absent and if electropalatography is used, these labels can easily be used alongside this instrumental technique. Therapy will follow the customary Metaphon stages and it will not be necessary to make adaptations at Phase 1 and Phase 2 Word Level apart from referring to production at Phase 2 if this is thought necessary.

Is Metaphon therapy successful with cleft palate children? An audit of 100 children with phoneme specific velopharyngeal incompetence (Harland and Albery, in preparation) suggests that children for whom articulation therapy was supplemented with Metaphon, as described above, achieved better generalisation to everyday speech than those who received articulation therapy alone. This audit was not a controlled study of therapeutic effectiveness, however, and the impression of better generalisation rests on subjective clinical opinion. There were probably many uncontrolled variables influencing response to therapy within this large group of children. There are plans to carry out systematic evaluation of this approach to therapy in the near future and we look forward to the results from this investigation.

Some Swedish children with cleft palate have also been treated using Metaphon principles with some success (Hellquist and Nyberg, personal communications) but we have no information about the nature of modifications, if any, that were made to Metaphon for these children. One child who used glottal substitution for all alveolar and velar sounds is reported as using alveolar plosives in all word positions after seven therapy sessions. She was also said to show marked improvement in the use of velar plosives and some change in the use of fricatives within the same time period. A second child eliminated stopping of fricatives after five therapy sessions. Although we have no experimental evidence so far the clinical impressions of the usefulness of Metaphon with this group of children, from both Britain and Sweden, should encourage exploration of using this type of therapy.

We do, of course, accept that many of the activities we use in Metaphon, including the strategies that we have suggested for those with congenital hearing loss, are not exclusive to Metaphon. What we do believe to be specific to Metaphon are the ways in which these strategies are used, within a framework where the goals and purpose of treatment are carefully specified and made explicit to the client. In the preceding paragraphs we have outlined some ways in which our methods might be adapted and employed with other client groups. It is part of our philosophy to encourage such experimentation in the general pursuit of a dynamic approach to the treatment of communication disorders. In our introduction, we said that this book marked the current state of our particular approach to the assessment and remediation of phonological disorder. We would stress that this is not a culmination, an end product, but a staging post and we hope our suggestions for wider application are taken in this spirit.

Metaphon in Other Languages

We have seen that Metaphon can be modified and used successfully with children with a variety of different problems as well as those with specifically disordered phonology. We end this chapter by looking at whether Metaphon can be adapted for languages other than English. We have information from Sweden, Wales and Holland.

The Swedish Experience

The following information about the use of Metaphon in Sweden comes from Britt Hellquist and Britta Eriksson. A critical evaluation of Metaphon from the Swedish perspective can be found in Nettelbladt (in press). Metaphon is widely practised in Sweden and is reported to be part of the basic training of all speech therapy students in the country. The approach has been the subject of papers published in Swedish and the 'Swedish Metafon Box' (Hellquist, 1992), which contains assessment and therapy material for use with Swedish children.

It was not difficult to transfer the Metaphon approach for use with the Swedish phonological system. The simplifying processes that occur in Swedish, are reported by Swedish therapists to be similar both in type and occurrence to those that occur in English, so no modifications were required to the therapy apart from translating it into another language.

In Sweden, as in Britain, Metaphon is used mainly with pre-school children with disordered phonology. Because children do not start school in Sweden until 7;0 tolerance of pronunciation errors is described as 'rather generous' and therapy tends not to be introduced for this group until around 4;6. Most Swedish recipients of Metaphon therefore are aged between 4;6 and 7, although the approach has been used with some phonologically disordered children as young as 3;6 and others as old as 13. The approach has also been used with Swedish children who have learning difficulties, hearing impairment or cleft palate.

Although there has not, to our knowledge, been any large scale systematic evaluation of Metaphon in Sweden, the rapid and widespread adoption of the approach is some testimony to its success there. But why has it been so successful? Undoubtedly the similarity between the phonological systems of Swedish and English speaking children was a factor in its success and it was also fortunate that the first Swedish academics and therapists who were introduced to Metaphon were excellent ambassadors for the approach. It is also possible that the child centred, discovery learning approach that is so central to Metaphon has a particular appeal because it is in sympathy with the Vygotskian view of the relationship between thought and language, which is very familiar to Swedish therapists. Nettelbladt (in press) suggests the possibility of interpreting Metaphon within a wider framework which includes theories coming from this tradition.

The Welsh Experience

Some therapists who use Metaphon with English speaking children have also been making attempts to adapt Metaphon for Welsh speaking children. We are grateful to Olwen Rees for exploring the possibilities of Metaphon in Welsh and providing us with the following information.

There are of course no language barriers to general adoption of the basic learning principles of the approach, that is, increasing metalinguistic awareness and encouraging reflection and active participation by the children. But there do appear to be major linguistic obstacles to employing the customary Metaphon procedures in a structured approach when treating Welsh speaking children. These are: the nature of the language itself and the lack of information about both the development of the Welsh phonological system and patterns of impaired phonological development.

Welsh has a similar sound system to English with the additional consonants of ‖ /ɬ/; ch, /χ/ and rh, /r̥/. (Ball and Jones, 1984). The phonotactic rules are also similar but not identical. The major difference between Welsh and English is that Welsh, in common with all Celtic languages, has both base forms and secondary forms. These secondary forms are mutations, or alterations, to the initial consonants of words in certain grammatical contexts. There are three different types of mutations each of which involves several different consonants. It is not appropriate to look in any detail at these mutations and which consonants are affected by each one but we will look at what might happen to mutations of /k/ to illustrate the complexity of this aspect of Welsh in the production of the word 'cadair' (chair). The base sound /k/ would change to /g/, 'ngh' or /c/ depending on the pronoun which preceded it as in – 'ei gadair' (his chair) 'fy **ngh**adair' (my chair) or 'ei chadair' (her chair).

Because there is no standardised information available about the development of the sound system in Welsh it is not known when sounds are expected to develop or when the mutations are incorporated into the sound system or whether they influence the base forms in any way.

Standardised data is difficult to compile because of factors which will variously influence the systems of individual children. For example, the systems of Welsh monoglot children, as in other languages, will be influenced by accent and the area of Wales they come from. Welsh monoglot children appear to present with different patterns to bilingual Welsh/English speakers, but this cannot be substantiated because of the lack of systematic investigation. In addition, most children by the age of four are exposed to two languages to some degree so this may also affect the later stages of development. Lack of knowledge about Welsh phonological development and the influence exerted by these other potential influencing factors makes it difficult to determine, particularly in the younger child, the nature and extent of phonological difficulties and as a consequence plan a systematic programme of therapy.

Despite the lack of standardised data, there is enough information available to suggest that there appears to be a fundamental difference in the development of the English and Welsh phonological systems. The information that is available on phonological development shows that on the whole Welsh monolingual children present with structural rather than systemic sound substitutions. This is especially true in the early acquisition stages, that is at the plosive and early fricative stage. Consistent 'stopping' and place errors are rare. The main feature in early Welsh phonological development is assimilation and consonant deletion. At a later stage of development there is much more similarity between the patterns observed in Welsh and English speaking children. Cluster simplification and reduction as well as liquid glide simplification would be similar as well as the usual /θ/→ [f] and /ð/ → [v] substitutions, and there are one or two other common sound substitutions specific to Welsh phonemes.

For the reasons stated above, the use of comprehensive structured

Metaphon programmes is not possible with Welsh speaking children. Therapists treating these children are not faced with the same patterns, and the common simplifying rules that are used by English speaking children are not clearly apparent in Welsh phonological development so the same therapy techniques are not going to be appropriate. There are some limited opportunities for using Metaphon activities for initial and final sound deletion, approximant substitutions and consonant cluster reduction, but even this is restricted because of the lack of therapeutically useful minimal pairs in Welsh.

So to summarise, it is not possible to emulate the Swedish experience and simply translate Metaphon into Welsh. The nature of the language and the lack of information about developmental patterns prevents the compilation of comprehensive structured Metaphon programmes for Welsh speaking children. The Welsh experience demonstrates the limitations of simple translation of a therapy approach formulated in one language to another language; limitations which may well apply to other Celtic language such as Gaelic. However, in this book it is appropriate to include the limitations as well as the positive aspects of Metaphon. We do believe, however, that it should be possible, when more is known about the phonological development of Welsh speaking children, to devise structured therapeutic techniques which might be quite different in appearance to Metaphon but will nevertheless be based on similar theoretical principles.

The Dutch Experience

Dutch speech therapists are also interested in using the Metaphon approach. Angela van den Oetelaar (personal communication) is currently adapting the Screening Assessment of the MRP for the Dutch language. There are currently no screening assessments available to assess the simplifying processes of Dutch speaking children. This version of the MRP is intended as a first step towards providing and assessing systematic Metaphon therapy for Dutch children with disordered phonology. Oetelaar expresses a hope that the Dutch MRP may in future be used as part of a cross linguistic study into the effects of Metaphon.

This is a task for the future, but this Dutch research together with the Swedish and Welsh interest in Metaphon is a promising start to the possibility of such an investigation.

In the final chapter we look at what else the future holds for the development of Metaphon.

Chapter 10
Conclusions

In this final chapter we review very briefly what we have attempted to do in this book and then go on to look at possible directions for the future of Metaphon.

Throughout this book we have attempted to translate theoretical ideas and constructs into practical application. We have endeavoured to demonstrate how, for one particular group of disordered children, application of theoretical concepts can enhance therapeutic practice for the benefit of both the client and practitioner. We looked first of all at the nature of phonological disorder concentrating particularly on the linguistic description of the disorder and in Chapter 3 we demonstrated how phonological analysis can inform therapeutic planning. We believe that our approach provides a good illustration of the way in which systematic analysis can be carried out by speech and language therapists, within a realistic time frame, to enhance the efficiency and effectiveness of intervention.

Our next focus was the concept that determines the therapeutic strategies in the Metaphon approach – linguistic awareness – and we then considered the learning theories which inform the therapeutic context. In Chapters 6 and 7 we went on to demonstrate how these concepts were combined in practice, and provided suggestions for treatment. In Chapter 8 we looked at the studies which have evaluated the Metaphon approach.

In Chapter 9 we explored the potential for using Metaphon in different clinical settings and with clients other than the specifically phonologically disordered. We hope that the information we have provided in Chapter 9 will give speech and language therapists additional help in using Metaphon with phonologically disordered children and encourage them to consider the possibility of applying our principles and therapy activities to other groups of children with communication problems.

The Future of Metaphon

In the first edition of this book we wrote that our primary focus for the future was to find out more about the effectiveness of Metaphon. There have been several developments since then. The application of Metaphon beyond its original conception and setting is something that has developed considerably in the last three or four years. We hope that this widening of application will continue. We saw in the last chapter that transferring the approach into other languages was not always straightforward. There has been interest in Metaphon from other European countries including Norway and we wait to hear of the experience of using Metaphon in this and other languages with interest. The development of Metaphon with cleft palate children is particularly interesting and demonstrates the possibility of making very specific modifications within the principles and structure of Metaphon for this client group. It is hoped that other therapists may be able to provide specific guidelines for adapting Metaphon for other specific groups of clients. We are for example frequently asked about the application of Metaphon to learning difficulties, and we have anecdotal evidence that some therapists do use this approach successfully with both children and adults. We anticipate that therapists will continue to investigate the use of Metaphon beyond the specific phonologically disordered population, and, where possible, carry out systematic evaluation of response to this therapy.

Our own specific concern is with the core structure and application of Metaphon. We will look at this from two main directions: monitoring its general effectiveness and examining ways in which the approach can provide optimum benefit for the individual child in the clinical setting.

Chapter 8 touched on the progress we have made in assessing the application of Metaphon since we published the results of the first efficacy study. The early results from the second efficacy study are very promising, supporting the results of our original investigation. Metaphon continues to show that it is effective in bringing about phonological change beyond that which might be expected with maturation. The inclusion of non-treated control groups in the second investigation has been particularly valuable in highlighting the relative roles of therapy and maturation in phonological change and we have acquired new information about the progress of such change. The opportunity to assess and reassess the output phonology of the treated and untreated children in our study shows that development was not static, but undergoing continual change in both groups. Metaphon therapy appears to accelerate that change.

These first impressions, if they are confirmed when our data collection and analysis are completed, have implications for future treatment planning and provision. It is possible that targeting therapy on those processes where change is taking place spontaneously will be the most efficient and effective strategy. An important task, then, is to discover where spontaneous change is occurring. Detailed analysis of each child's phonological system becomes even more important in assisting us in this endeavour; close examination of the variability and the extent of application of simplifying processes would be particularly enlightening. It might also be appropriate to adopt different assessment policies, possibly administering an initial assessment and then readministering it a short time later before starting therapy. The time intervals between assessment and reassessment in the second efficacy study give an indication of how long this period might be. It should not be difficult to design a small research investigation to test out the possibilities we have suggested.

Before we leave this question of spontaneous phonological change it is appropriate to mention the implications our initial results have for interpreting and carrying out research into therapeutic effectiveness. They highlight the need to continue to investigate the relative roles of maturation and therapy in phonological change. In practical terms this means including untreated control groups and/or paying very careful attention to establishing reliable base lines before starting therapy. Studies which attribute change to the effects of therapy without these safeguards should be treated with caution.

The first results from the second efficacy study therefore have strengthened the justification for using the Metaphon approach and have provided us with information which may influence where we target therapy. This investigation has also enabled us to start addressing our second concern – exploring ways of making Metaphon optimally effective in the clinical setting for the individual child. One way of looking at this concern is through the second question addressed by this investigation which was to ask whether both phases of Metaphon were necessary to bring about phonological change. The original purpose behind this question was to find out how Metaphon worked. We had no way of knowing from our clinical work, or the first efficacy study, what aspects of Metaphon were crucial in bringing about phonological change and therefore what aspects we might have to change or emphasise in practical application.

Finding out why Metaphon is effective is also a basic theoretical concern. If we can obtain this information it may enhance our understanding of why some children have difficulties with phonological acquisition, a question which so far has not been satisfactorily answered. A first step in understanding why Metaphon works can also be made through exploring the relative contributions of the two phases of the approach.

Clinicians are increasingly asking, in the interests of efficiency and economy, whether both phases of Metaphon are required; see for instance Howard and Hesketh (1993). We are starting to get some answers to this question. Children in both treated groups in the second efficacy study, as we saw in Chapter 8, are showing greater phonological change than the non-treated children. But there is a tendency for Group 2 children to show more generalised change than Group 1 children, that is change is less likely to be restricted to the process that was targeted in therapy. Once again we have to be cautious about drawing inferences from what are very preliminary results but the indications seem to be that some children may only require the metaphonological knowledge provided in Phase 1 to start the process of change. We will not of course know, until we get further information from the children's therapists, whether change continues and whether these children over time will show the same generalisation patterns as those shown by Group 2 children.

So what are the clinical implications of this finding? We do not predict that it will lead to any radical changes in the general design of the Metaphon framework. In our view these results reinforce the importance of adapting therapy to suit the needs of individual children. Regular monitoring and constant observation of the children's responses to treatment will determine how long and in what ways a particular process should be targeted. In Chapter 7 we saw that different children spent different amounts of time in each phase of therapy. Some children will need more activities than others at each stage of Metaphon and some may need few or no activities at Phase 2, but this can only be determined by responding to each child's response to therapy. There may indeed be some children who require therapy that concentrates mainly on Phase 2 activities. The case of Mike (Example 4 in Chapter 3) can serve as an illustration of how individual needs can be determined. We saw that Mike tended to be rather resistant to therapy until Phase 2 activities were introduced. We do not believe that a satisfactory answer to this would be to abandon Phase 1 activities and focus only on communicative change; his comments and behaviour during therapy suggested he needed more information about the sounds he was having difficulty with. It is perhaps also important to stress here that the basic principles on which Metaphon is based are not compatible with just providing Phase 2 therapy. We do not believe that this would provide sufficient information, at least for most children, to enable them to make the required changes in their phonological output. Our own clinical experience and that of other therapists suggests that response to Metaphon is poor if children do not have explicit information about the sound system to draw upon. To return to Mike, it would perhaps have been helpful in his particular case if we had designed therapy activities for him which brought together Phase 1 and Phase 2 activities more closely, or simply introduced Phase 2 activities earlier to run alongside Phase 1 activities so that they reinforced each other more specifically and directly. It is of course easy to suggest possible changes with the benefit of hindsight and responding to the children's needs must always to an extent be a matter of trial and error. Perhaps we need to stress again, as we have done several times throughout this book, that Metaphon is essentially a rationale, a philosophy, and not a programme. Its strength lies in its flexibility. But the more children we treat using Metaphon the more skilled we become at tailoring it to individual needs.

Another factor in maximising the effectiveness of Metaphon is to see to what extent we can modify the therapeutic tasks we use in Metaphon to match the individual characteristics of each child. An important aspect of such modifications is the provision of guidelines for adapting Metaphon for sub-groups within the phonologically disordered population. We saw in Chapter 9, where we discussed possible adaptations for children with motor processing limitations, that a start has already been made in this direction. Establishing further guidelines will depend on determining further sub-groups. This can partly be accomplished by investigations which examine strengths and weaknesses in speech processing and partly by analysing children's responses to the various aspects of Metaphon therapy. One of the aims of the second efficacy study was to account for the different responses to Metaphon that we had found in our first investigation. The assessment measures we are currently using are designed to tell us something about the relationship between effectiveness and speech processing characteristics.

Information is also being collected about other individual child characteristics. A comparison of these results with response to therapy will also be helpful in determining how effective therapy might be for a particular client and what steps might be taken to increase potential effectiveness. One particular area of interest, which might have implications for a general modification of Metaphon for some children, is the question of cognitive style. If the measures of reflection and impulsivity that we are using show that this aspect of behaviour is found to have an influence on response to therapy, designing suitable therapy activities to meet individual differences along the reflection impulsivity continuum will be an exciting challenge for the future.

Finally in our discussion about the future of Metaphon we want to return to look at phonological processes. We have seen that for some children change is specific to the processes treated and for others it is much more general. We have suggested that some differences in response might be accounted for by individual child characteristics of various kinds but we have not yet considered whether different patterns of response might be associated with possible interrelationships between processes. Our current research will help to determine whether providing treatment for one process will lead to change in other processes. Such knowledge will help us to make predictions about the order in which processes should be targeted in the interests of efficient treatment.

We have looked at several factors which might affect response to Metaphon therapy and our discussion of the future of this approach has centred mainly on the need to discover what these factors are so that we can increase its efficiency and effectiveness. In some respects this is an impossible task; for each child there will be many factors which influence how he or she responds to Metaphon or indeed to any therapy or learning situation. At the moment we are able to say, as we did in the first edition, that for some children Metaphon may work because we have provided an appropriate learning environment which encourages them to experiment. For others we may have provided phonological knowledge which they previously lacked. Other children may have such knowledge but may not have used it to facilitate their own phonological development. So there are no simple answers and indeed we would not expect any. Metaphon continues to challenge its practitioners to understand the ways in which it effects phonological change.

In the introductory chapter we said that this book represented not an end point but a rest along the way in finding out more about the link between phonological development and linguistic awareness, the foundation of our therapy approach. One thing we do know, that is worth restating, is that we cannot simply equate delayed phonological development with poor metalinguistic ability. We saw in Chapter 4 that phonologically disordered children as a group have poorer linguistic awareness than their normally developing peers. But we also saw that there were considerable individual differences between children and that some phonologically disordered children displayed very good metalinguistic ability. If we can discover more about why children respond to a treatment approach such as Metaphon it will perhaps help us to increase our understanding of phonological disorder and development.

Our primary aim throughout this book has been to produce a resource which can be used for practical application. Our secondary, less tangible aim has been to present this practical tool within a framework of theory, as a contribution to the provision of principled therapy and to progress the development of a science of intervention. We hope that we have succeeded to some extent in both aims so that readers will not only be encouraged to try out our methods but will also think more deeply about the process of treatment for people who have difficulties with communication.

References

Abbs, J.H. and Kennedy, J.G. (1982). Neurophysiological processes of speech movement and control. In: J.L. Lass, L.V. McReynolds, J.L. Northern, and D.E. Yoder, (Eds.), *Speech Language and Hearing*, Vol. 1. Philadelphia: W.B. Saunders Co.

Aitchison, J. (1987). *Words in the Mind: An Introduction to the Mental Lexicon*. Oxford: Blackwell.

Aitchison, J. and Chiat, S. (1981). Natural phonology or natural memory? The interaction between phonological processes and recall mechanisms. *Language and Speech* 24, 311–326.

Anthony, A., Bogle, D., Ingram, T.T.S.I. and McIsaac, M.W. (1971). *The Edinburgh Articulation Test*. Edinburgh: Livingstone.

Ball, M.J. and Jones, G.E. (Eds.) (1984). *Welsh Phonology*. Cardiff: University of Wales Press.

Barton, D., Miller, R. and Macken, M.A. (1980). Do children treat clusters as one unit or two? *Papers and Reports on Child Language Development* 18, 105–137. Stanford: Stanford University Press.

Berko, J. and Brown, R. (1960). Psycholinguistic research methods. In: P. Mussen (Ed.), *Handbook of Research Methods in Child Development*. New York: Wiley.

Bernhardt, B. and Gilbert, J. (1992). Applying linguistic theory to speech–language pathology: the case for non-linear phonology. *Clinical Linguistics and Phonetics*, 6, 123–145.

Beveridge, M. and Griffiths, R. (1983). The social context of learning in the classroom. In: K. Wheldall and R. Riding (Eds.), *Psychological Aspects of Learning and Teaching*. London: Croom Helm.

Bird, J. and Bishop, D. (1992). Perception and awareness of phonemes in phonologically impaired children. *European Journal of Disorders of Communication*, 27, 289–311.

Bishop, D. and Edmundson, A. (1987). Language impaired 4 year olds: distinguishing transient from persistent impairment. *Journal of Speech and Hearing Disorders* 52, 156–173.

Bishop, D. and Rosenbloom, L. (1987). Childhood language disorders: classification and overview. In: W. Yule and M. Rutter (Eds.), *Language Development and Disorders*. Oxford: Blackwell Scientific.

Bowerman, M. (1978). Words and sentences: uniformity, individual variation and shifts over time in patterns of acquisition. In: F. Minifie and L. Lloyd (Eds.),

Communicative and Cognitive Abilities – Early Behavioural Assessment.
Baltimore: University Park Press.

Bradley, L. and Bryant, P.E. (1978). Difficulties in auditory organisation as a possible cause of reading backwardness. *Nature* 271, 746–747.

Bradley, L. and Bryant, P.E. (1983). Categorising sounds and learning to read – a causal connection. *Nature* 301, 419–421.

Bruner, J. (1983). *Child's Talk. Learning to Use Language*. Oxford: University Park Press.

Bryant, P.E. and Bradley, L. (1985). *Children's Reading Problems*. Oxford: Basil Blackwell.

Cazden, C. (1972). *Child Language and Education*. New York: Holt, Rinehart & Winston.

Cazden, C. (1976). Play with language and metalinguistic awareness, One dimension of language experience. In: J.S. Bruner, A. Jolly and K. Sylva (Eds.) *Play – Its Role in Development and Evolution*. Harmondsworth: Penguin Books.

Cazden, C.B. (1983). Play with language and metalinguistic awareness: one dimension of language experience. In: M. Donaldson, R. Grieve and C. Pratt (Eds.), *Early Childhood Development and Education*. Oxford: Blackwell.

Chaney, C. (1992). Language development, metalinguistic skills and print awareness in 3 year old children. *Applied Psycholinguistics* 13, 485–514.

Chiat, S. (1979). The role of the word in phonological development. *Linguistics* 17, 591–610.

Chiat, S. (1983). Why Mikey's right and my key's wrong: the significance of stress and word boundaries in a child's output system. *Cognition* 14, 275–300.

Chukovsky, K. (1968). *From Two to Five*. Berkeley and Los Angeles: University of California Press.

Clark, R. (1983). How do children learn to talk? In: K. Wheldall and R. Riding (Eds.), *Psychological Aspects of Learning and Teaching*. London: Croom Helm

Clark, E.V. (1978). Awareness of language: some evidence from what children say and do. In: A. Sinclair, R. J. Jarvella and W. J. M. Levelt (Eds.), *The Child's Conception of Language*. Berlin: Springer Verlag.

Clark, E. V. and Andersen, E. S. (1979). Spontaneous repairs: awareness in the process of acquiring language. *Papers and Reports on Child Language Development* 16, 1–12. Stanford: Stanford University.

Code, C. (1985). Investigating the efficacy of treatment with a simple ABA single-case design. *Bulletin of The College of Speech Therapists*, 394, February.

Coltheart, M. (1989). Aphasia therapy research: a single-case approach. In: C. Code and D. J. Muller (Eds.), *Aphasia Therapy* (Second Edition). London: Whurr.

Constable, C. M. (1986). The application of scripts in the organisation of language intervention contexts. In: K. Nelson (Ed.), *Event Knowledge. Structure and Function in Development*. Hillsdale, New Jersey: Lawrence Erlbaum Associates.

Crystal, D. (1987). Towards a bucket theory of language disability; taking account of interaction between linguistic levels. *Clinical Linguistics and Phonetics* 1, 7–22.

Dean, E.C. and Howell, J. (1986). Developing linguistic awareness: a theoretically based approach to phonological disorders. *British Journal of Disorders of Communication* 21, 223–238.

Dean, E.C., Howell, J., Hill, A. and Waters, D. (1990). *Metaphon Resource Pack*. Windsor, Berks: NFER Nelson.

Dean, E.C., Anderson, C. and Waters, D.M. (1992). The Metaphon approach to therapy: implications for children with articulatory as well as phonological constraints. *Bulletin of the College of Speech and Language Therapists*, 486, 12.

Dean, E.C., Howell, J., Waters, D.M. and Reid, J. (in press). Metaphon: a metalinguistic approach to the treatment of phonological disorder in children. *Clinical Linguistics and Phonetics*.

Deutsch, S.E. (1984). Oral stereognosis. In: C. Code and M.J. Ball (Eds.), *Experimental Clinical Phonetics*. Beckenham: Croom Helm.

de Villiers, P.A. and de Villiers, J.G. (1972). Early judgements of syntactic and semantic acceptability by children. *Journal of Psycholinguistic Research* 1, 299–310.

Dinnsen, D.A. (1984). Methods and empirical issues in analyzing functional misarticulation. In: M. Elbert, D.A. Dinnsen and G. Weismer (Eds.), *Phonological Theory and the Misarticulating Child*. ASHA Monographs 22. Rockville, Maryland: American Speech-Language-Hearing Association.

Dodd, B. and Iacano, T. (1989). Phonological disorders in chldren: changes in phonological processes durng treatment. *British Journal of Disorders of Communication* 24, 333–351.

Dowker, A. (1989). Rhyme and alliteration in children's poems. *Journal of Child Language* 16, 181–202.

Dunn, C. and Davis. B, (1983). Phonological process occurrence in phonologically disordered children. *Applied Psycholinguistics* 4, 187–207.

Dunn, L. M., Dunn, L., Whetton, C. and Pintilie, D. (1982). *British Picture Vocabulary Scales*. Windsor: NFER Nelson.

Edwards, M., Brown, D., Cape, J. and Foreman, D. (1984). *Criteria for selection of children for speech therapy*. Unpublished report of the Department of Health and Social Services.

Fox, B. and Routh, D. K. (1975). Analyzing spoken language into words, syllables and phonemes: a developmental study. *Journal of Psycholinguistic Research* 4, 331–342.

Gardner, H. (1989). An investigation of maternal interaction with phonologically disordered children as compared to two groups of normally developing children. *British Journal of Disorders of Communication* 24, 41–59.

Garton, A. and Pratt, C. (1989). *Learning to be Literate. The Development of Spoken and Written Language*. Oxford: Blackwell.

Garvey, C. (1977). Play with language and speech. In: S. Ervin-Tripp and C. Mitchell-Kernan (Eds.), *Child Discourse*. New York: Academic Press.

Gathercole, S.E. and Baddeley, A.D. (1993). *Working Memory and Language*. Hove: Lawrence Erlbaum Associates.

Gathercole, S.E., Willis, C., Baddeley, A. and Emslie, H. (1994). The children's test of nonword repetition: a test of phonological working memory. *Memory* 4, 103–127.

Gibbon, F. and Grunwell, P. (1990). Specific developmental language learning difficulties. In: P Grunwell (Ed.), *Developmental Speech Disorders: Clinical Issues and Practical Implications*. Edinburgh: Churchill Livingstone

Gleitman, L.R., Gleitman, H. and Shipley, E.F. (1972). The emergence of the child as a grammarian. *Cognition* 1, 137–164.

Gombert, J.E. (1992). *Metalinguistic Development*. London: Harvester Wheatsheaf.

Goswami, U. and Bryant, P.E. (1990). *Phonological Skills and Learning to Read*. Hove: Lawrence Erlbaum.

Grunwell, P. (1981). *The Nature of Phonological Disability in Children*. London: Academic Press.

Grunwell, P. (1983). Phonological therapy: premises, principles and procedures.

XIX Congress of IALP. August, University of Edinburgh.

Grunwell, P. (1985). *Phonological Assessment of Child Speech: PACS*. Windsor: NFER-Nelson.

Grunwell, P. (1987). *Clinical Phonology* (2nd Edition). London: Croom Helm.

Grunwell, P. (1990). *Developmental Speech Disorders: Clinical Issues and Practical Implications*. Edinburgh: Churchill Livingstone.

Hambrecht, G. and Panagos, J.M. (1980). Phonological influences on children's sentence repetition. *Human Communication* 5, 69–74.

Harland K. and Albery, L. (In preparation) Management of 100 cases of phoneme specific nasality – a two centre audit. To appear in: *British Journal of Plastic Surgery*.

Hartman, E. and Haarvind, H. (1981). Mothers as teachers and their children as learners: a study of the influence of social interaction on cognitive development. In: W. P. Robinson (Ed.), *Communication in Development*. London: Academic Press.

Hellquist, B. (1992). *Metafon på Svenska*. Löddköpinge: Pedagogisk Design.

Henry, C.E. (1990). The development of oral diadochokinesia and non-linguistic rhythmic skills in normal and speech disordered young children. *Clinical Linguistics and Phonetics* 4, 121–137.

Hewlett, N. (1990). The processes of speech production and speech development. In: P. Grunwell (Ed.), *Developmental Speech Disorders: Clinical Issues and Practical Implications*. Edinburgh: Churchill Livingstone.

Hodson, B.W. (1980). *The Assessment of Phonological Processes*. Danvill, Illinois: Interstate Printers and Publishers.

Howard, L. and Hesketh, A. (1993). Metaphon; from effectiveness to efficiency. *Bulletin of the College of Speech and Language Therapists* 500, 6–7.

Howell, J. (1989). *The Metalinguistic Awareness of Phonologically Disordered and Normally Developing Children: a Comparative Study*. Unpublished PhD Thesis: University of Newcastle Upon Tyne.

Howell, J. and Dean, E. (1987). "I think that's a noisy sound": reflection and learning in the therapeutic situation. *Child Language Teaching and Therapy* 3, 259–266.

Howell, J. and McCartney, E. (1990). Approaches to remediation. In: P. Grunwell (Ed.), *Developmental Speech Disorders: Clinical Issues and Practical Implications*. Edinburgh: Churchill Livingstone.

Ingram, D. (1976). *Phonological Disability in Children*. London: Edward Arnold.

Ingram, D. (1981). *Procedures for the Phonological Analysis of Children's Language*. Baltimore: University Park Press.

Ingram, D. (1986). Phonological development: production. In: P. Fletcher and M. Garman (Eds.), *Language Acquisition: Studies in First Language Development* (2nd edition). Cambridge: Cambridge University Press.

Iwamura, O. (1980). *The Verbal Games of Pre-school Children*. London: Croom Helm.

Kamhi, A.G., Friemoth-Lee, R. and Nelson, L.K. (1985). Word, syllable and sound awareness in language disordered children. *Journal of Speech and Hearing Disorders* 50, 207–212.

Kiparsky, P. and Menn, L. (1977). On the acquisition of phonology. In: J. MacNamara (Ed.), *Language Learning and Thought*. New York: Academic Press.

Kirk, S.A., McCarthy, J.J. and Kirk, W.D. (1968). *Illinois Test of Psycholinguistic Abilities* (Revised edition). Illinois: University of Illinois Press.

Kuczaj, S.A. (1983). *Crib Speech and Language Play*. New York: Springer-Verlag.

Leonard, L.B.(1973).The nature of disordered articulation. *Journal of Speech and Hearing Disorders* 38, 156–161.

Leonard, L. B. (1985). Unusual and subtle phonological behaviour in the speech of phonological disordered children. *Journal of Speech and Hearing Disorders* 50, 4–13.

Liberman, I.Y., Shankweiler, D., Fischer, F.W. and Carter, B. (1974). Explicit phoneme and syllable segmentation in the young chld. *Journal of Experimental Child Psychology* 18, 201–212.

Locke, J. (1980). The inference of speech perception in the phonologically disordered child: Part I. *Journal of Speech and Hearing Disorders* 45, 431–444.

Lucariello, J., Kyratzis, A. and Engel, S. (1986). Event representations, context and language. In: K. Nelson (Ed.), *Event Knowledge. Structure and Function in Development*. Hillsdale, New Jersey: Lawrence Erlbaum Associates.

McCartney, E. (1981). The response of speech disordered children to requests for clarification. *British Journal of Disorders of Communication* 16, 147–158.

Maccoby, E.E., Dowley, E.M., Hagan, J. and Degerman, R. (1965). Activity level and intellectual functioning in normal pre-school children. *Child Development* 36, 761–770.

Macken, M. (1980). The child's lexical representation: The "puzzle-puddle-pickle" evidence. *Journal of Linguistics* 16, 1–19.

Macken, M. and Ferguson, C.A. (1983). Cognitive aspects of phonological development: model evidence and issues. In: K.E. Nelson (Ed.), *Children's Language*, Vol 4. Hillsdale, New Jersey: Lawrence Erlbaum Associates.

Magnusson, E. (1983). The phonology of language disordered children: production, perception and awareness. *Travaux de l'Institut De Linguistique de Lund* xvii: Lund: CWK Gleerup.

Magnusson, E. (1991) Metalinguistic awareness in phonologically disordered children. In: M.S. Yavas (Ed.), *Phonological Disorders in Children: Theory Research and Practice*. London: Routledge.

Magnusson, E. and Naucler, K. (1987). Language disordered and normally speaking children's development of spoken and written language: preliminary results from a longitudinal study. *RUVL* 16, Uppsala University: Department of Linguistics.

Menn, L. (1976). Evidence for an interactionist-discovery theory of child phonology. *Papers and Reports on Child Language Development* 12, 169–177. Stanford: Stanford University.

Menyuk, P., Liebergott, J. and Schultz M. (1986). Predicting Phonologial Development. In: B. Linblom and R. Zetterstrom (Eds.) *Precursors of Early Speech*. Werner-Gren International Symposium Series, Vol. 44. London: Macmillan.

Menyuk, P., Menn, L. and Silber, P. (1986). Phonological development: production. In: P. Fletcher and M. Garman (Eds.), *Language Acquisition (2nd Edition)*. Cambridge: Cambridge University Press.

Mogford, K. and Bishop, D. (1988). Five questions about language acquisition considered in the light of exceptional circumstances. In: D. Bishop and K. Mogford (Eds.), *Language Development in Exceptional Circumstances*. Edinburgh: Churchill Livingstone.

Moss, F.A. (1985). *A Theoretical and Experimental Investigation of the Nature of Phonological and Phonetic Processes in the Speech of Children with Phonological Disorders*. Unpublished M.Phil Thesis, Council for National Academic Awards.

Naucler, K. and Magnusson, E. (1984). *Language disordered children's reading and spelling*. Paper presented at the 7th World Congress of Applied Linguistics. Brussels, Belgium: August 5–10.

Nelson, K. (1986). Event knowledge and cognitive development. In: K. Nelson (Ed.), *Event Knowledge. Structure and Function in Development*. Hillsdale, New Jersey: Lawrence Erlbaum Associates.

Nettelbladt, U. (in press) The Metaphon approach to phonological therapy from a Swedish perspective. *Clinical Linguistics and Phonetics*.

Panagos, J.M., Quine, M.E.and Klich, R.J. (1979). Syntactic and phonological influences on children's articulation. *Journal of Speech and Hearing Research* 22, 841–848.

Perret-Clermont, A.N. and Schubauer-Leoni, M. (1981). Conflict and co-operation as opportunities for learning. In: W. P. Robinson (Ed.), *Communication in Development*. London: Academic Press.

Peters, A.M. (1983). *The Units of Language Acquisition*. Cambridge: Cambridge University Press.

Pratt, C. and Grieve, R. (1984a). The development of metalinguistic awareness: an introduction. In: W. E. Tunmer, C. Pratt and M. L. Herriman (Eds.), *Metalinguistic Awareness in Children. Theory, Research and Implications*. Berlin: Springer-Verlag.

Pratt, C. and Grieve, R. (1984b). Metalinguistic awareness and cognitive development. In: W.E. Tunmer, C. Pratt and M.L. Herriman (Eds.), *Metalinguistic Awareness in Children. Theory, Research and Implications*. Berlin: Springer-Verlag.

Rapin, I. and Allen, D. (1983). Developmental language disorders: nosological considerations. In: V. Kirk (Ed.), *Neuropsychology of Language, Reading and Spelling*. New York: Academic Press.

Read, C. (1978). Children's awareness of language with emphasis on sound systems. In: A. Sinclair, R. J. Jarvella and W. J. Levelt (Eds.), *The Child's Conception of Language*. Berlin: Springer Verlag.

Reid, J. (1989). *Awareness of Phonemes, Phonological Disorder and the Acquisition of Literacy in Children*. Unpublished MA dissertation, University of Reading.

Reid, J., Grieve, R., Dean, E.C., Donaldson, M.L. and Howell, J. (1993). Linguistic awareness in young children. In: J. Clibbens and B. Pendleton (Eds.), *Proceedings of Child Language Seminar, University of Plymouth, 1993*. 255–274.

Reynell, J.K. (1977). *Reynell Developmental Language Scales (Revised)*. Windsor: NFER.

Reynolds, J. (1990) Abnormal vowel patterns in phonological disorder: some data and a hypothesis. *British Journal of Disorders of Communication* 25, 115–148.

Robinson, E.J. and Robinson, W.P. (1983a). Ways of reacting to communication failure in relation to the developments of the child's understanding about verbal communication. In: M. Donaldson, R. Grieve and C Pratt (Eds.), *Early Childhood Development and Education*. Oxford: Blackwell.

Robinson, E.J. and Robinson, W.P. (1983b). Children's uncertainty about the interpretation of ambiguous messages. *Journal of Experimental Child Psychology*, 36, 81–96.

Robinson, E.J. and Robinson, W.P. (1985). Teaching children about verbal referential communication. *International Journal of Behavioural Development*, 8, 285–289.

Schuele, C.M. and Van Kleek, A. (1987). Precursors to literacy: assessment and intervention. *Topics in Language Disorders* 7, 32–44.

Schwartz, R.G. (1991). Interactions among language components in phonological development and disorders. In: M.S. Yavas (Ed.), *Phonological Disorders in Children: Theory Research and Practice*. London: Routledge.

Shriberg, L.D. and Kwiatkowski, J. (1980). *Natural Process Analysis*. New York: John Wiley.

Shriberg, L.D., Kwiatkowski, J., Best, S., Hengst, J. and Terselic-Weber, B. (1986). Characteristics of children with phonologic disorders of unknown origin. *Journal of Speech and Hearing Disorders* 51, 140–161.

Sinclair, A., Jarvella, R.J. and Levelt, W.M.J. (1978). *The Child's Conception of Language*. Berlin: Springer-Verlag.

Smit, A.B. and Bernthal, J.E. (1983). Performance of articulation disordered children on language and perception measures. *Journal of Speech and Hearing Research* 26, 124–136.

Smith, N.V. (1973). *The Acquisition of Phonology: A Case Study*. Cambridge: Cambridge University Press.

Snow, C.E., Dubber, C. and de Blauw, A. (1982). Routines in mother–child interaction. In: I. Feagans and D.C. Farran (Eds.), *The Language of Children Reared in Poverty*. New York: Academic Press.

Snowling, M.J. (Ed.) (1985). *Children's Written Language Difficulties: Assessment and Management*. Windsor, Berks: NFER-Nelson.

Snowling M., Chiat, S. and Hume, C. (1991). Words, nonwords and phonological processes: Some comments on Gathercole, Willis, Emslie and Baddeley. *Applied Psycholinguistics* 12, 369–373.

Stackhouse, J. (1985). Segmentation, speech and spelling difficulties. In: M.J. Snowling (Ed.), *Children's Written Language Difficulties*. Windsor, Berks: NFER-Nelson.

Stackhouse, J. and Snowling, M. (1983). Segmentation and spelling in children with speech disorders. In: M. Edwards (Ed.), *Proceedings of XIX Congress of the International Association of Logopaedics and Phoniatrics*. London: College of Speech Therapists, 282–287.

Stackhouse, J. and Wells, B. (1993). Psycholinguistic assessment of developmental speech disorders. *European Journal of Disorders of Communication* 28, 331–348.

Stampe, D. (1979). *A Dissertation on Natural Phonology*. New York: Garland.

Stoel-Gammon, C. and Dunn, C. (1985). *Normal and Disordered Phonology in Children*. Baltimore: University Park Press.

Straight, H.S. (1980). Auditory versus articulatory phonological processes and their development in children. In: G.H. Yeni-Komshian, J.F. Kavanagh and C.A. Ferguson (Eds.), *Child Phonology Volume 1: Production*. New York: Academic Press.

Strange, R.W. and Broen, P.A. (1980). Perception and production of approximant consonants by 3-year-olds: a first study. In: G. Yeni-Komshian, J.F. Kavanagh and C. A. Ferguson (Eds.), *Child Phonology Volume 2: Perception*. New York: Academic Press.

Supple, M. de Montfort (1983). Auditory perceptual function in relation to phonological development. *British Journal of Audiology* 17, 59–68.

Tough, J. (1982). Teachers can create enabling environments for children and then children will learn. In: L. Reagans and D.C. Farran (Eds.), *The Language of Children Reared in Poverty*. New York: Academic Press.

Treiman, R. (1985). Onsets and rimes as units of spoken syllables. *Journal of Experimental Child Psychology* 39, 161–181.

Treiman, R. (1994). Distributional constraints and syllable structure in English. *Journal of Phonetics* 16, 221–229.

Tunmer, W.E. and Herriman, M.L.(1984). The development of metalinguistic awareness: A conceptual overview. In: W.E. Tunmer, C. Pratt and M.L. Herriman (Eds.) *Metalinguistic Awareness in Children: Theory, Research and Implications*. Berlin: Springer Verlag.

Vance, M. (in press). "Sock the wock the pit-pat pock" – children's responses to measures of rhyming ability. To appear in: *Proceedings of the Child Language Seminar, Bangor, 1994* and *National Hospital College of Speech Sciences Work in Progress, 1994*.

Waters, D. (1992). *An Investigation of Motor Control for Speech in Phonologically Delayed Children, Normally Developing Children and Adults*. Unpublished PhD Thesis: Council for National Academic Awards.

Waterson, N. (1981). A tentative developmental model of phonological representation. In: T. Myers, J. Laver and J. Anderson (Eds.) *The Cognitive Representation of Speech*. Amsterdam: North Holland Publishing Company.

Waterson, N. (1987). *Prosodic Phonology. The Theory and Its Application to Language Acquisition and Speech Processing*. Newcastle Upon Tyne: Grevatt & Grevatt.

Wechsler, D. (1967). *Wechsler Pre-school and Primary Scale of Intelligence*. New York: Psychological Corporation.

Weiner, F. (1979). *Phonological Process Analysis*. Baltimore: University Park Press.

Weiner, F.F. and Ellis, C. (1980). *Tolerance for homonymy: a factor in children's misarticulation*. Paper presented at American Speech-Language-Hearing Association Congress, Detroit.

Weiner, F.F. and Ostrowski, A. (1979). Effects of listener uncertainty on articulatory inconsistency. *Journal of Speech and Hearing Disorders* 44, 487–493.

Weir, R.H. (1962). *Language in the Crib*. The Hague: Mouton.

Wells, C.G. (1978). What makes for successful language development? In: R. Campbell and P. Smith (Eds.), *Advances in the Psychology of Language (Volume 2)*. New York: Plenum.

Winitz, H. (1969). *Articulatory Acquisition and Behavior*. New York: Appleton Century Crofts.

Wright, J.C., Gaughan, D.J. and McClanachan, R. (1978). *Kansas Reflection Impulsivity Scale for Pre-Schoolers*. Kansas Centre for Research in Early Childhood Education, University of Kansas.

Zhurova, L.Y. (1973). Development of analysis of words into their sounds by pre-school children. In: C.A. Ferguson and D.I. Slobin (Eds.), *Studies of Child Language Development*. New York: Holt, Rinehart & Winston.

Index

Author Index